AF412904

Home Dialysis in Japan

Contributions to Nephrology

Vol. 177

Series Editor

Claudio Ronco Vicenza

Home Dialysis in Japan

Contemporary Status

Volume Editor

Hiromichi Suzuki Saitama

48 figures, 16 in color, and 25 tables, 2012

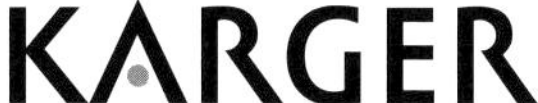

Basel · Freiburg · Paris · London · New York · New Delhi · Bangkok · Beijing · Tokyo · Kuala Lumpur · Singapore · Sydney

Contributions to Nephrology

(Founded 1975 by Geoffrey M. Berlyne)

Hiromichi Suzuki
Department of Nephrology
Community Health Science Center
38 Morohonngo, Moroyama cho
Irumagun, 350-0495, Saitama
Japan

Library of Congress Cataloging-in-Publication Data

Home dialysis in Japan : contemporary status / volume editor, Hiromichi
Suzuki.
     p. ; cm. -- (Contributions to nephrology, ISSN 0302-5144 ; v. 177)
  Includes bibliographical references and index.
  ISBN 978-3-318-02109-7 (hard cover : alk. paper) -- ISBN 978-3-318-02110-3
(e-ISBN)
  I. Suzuki, Hiromichi, M.D. II. Series: Contributions to nephrology ; v.
177. 0302-5144
  [DNLM: 1. Hemodialysis, Home--Japan. W1 CO778UN v.177 2012 / WJ 378]

  617.4'610952--dc23
                                        2012009677

Bibliographic Indices. This publication is listed in bibliographic services, including Current Contents® and Index Medicus.

© Copyright 2012 by S. Karger AG, P.O. Box, CH–4009 Basel (Switzerland)
www.karger.com
Printed in Germany on acid-free and non-aging paper (ISO 9706) by Bosch Druck, Ergolding
ISSN 0302–5144
e-ISSN 1662–2782
ISBN 978–3–318–02109–7
e-ISBN 978–3–318–02110–3

Contents

Home Hemodialysis

Preface

The *Overview of Regular Dialysis Treatment in Japan* showed that in 2010, approximately 300,000 people with end-stage renal disease (ESRD) required renal replacement therapy. More than 95% of these patients undergo in-center hemodialysis, which is typically delivered three times a week. Dialysis therapy was originally introduced to support ambulatory patients able to work and participate in social activities. However, in recent years a large component of the patients receiving dialysis therapy were diabetic and elderly, which caused a drastic change in dialysis therapy. The aim of dialysis therapy was altered to prolong life without consideration of quality of life. In Japan after World War II, westernization had a profound impact on the diet and lifestyle of the people. In this situation, some patients wished to have dialysis therapy (peritoneal dialysis (PD) and home hemodialysis HHD) at home based on individual preferences. Since dialysis therapy was introduced, machines and solutions used in dialysis therapy have been greatly improved in Japan, extending the lifespan of patients receiving dialysis therapy to two to three times longer than that of other countries. The ingenuity and creative energy of the Japanese for producing new machines and systems for patients receiving PD and HHD may contribute to new developments and progression of home dialysis therapy in the world.

This book is intended to acquaint the reader of the fruits of recent progress made in PD and HHD therapy in Japan.

Hiromichi Suzuki, Saitama

Suzuki H (ed): Home Dialysis in Japan.
Contrib Nephrol. Basel, Karger, 2012, vol 177, pp 1–2

Introduction

Allan J. Collins

Chronic Disease Research Group, University of Minnesota, Minneapolis, USA

The Growing Burden of Dialysis Treatment in Japan and the United States: Is It Time for More Diversification to Home Treatment Modalities?

The growing number of dialysis patients in Japan and the USA has placed a growing strain on the healthcare budgets of both countries. In Japan, end-stage renal disease (ESRD) treatment accounts for 4.5% of the healthcare budget, a greater percentage than in the USA. The challenges for both countries center on the ever-expanding population with kidney failure, the improving survival of the prevalent population and the expanding expenditures for new treatments for anemia, bone and mineral disease, vascular disease and diabetes. In Japan, the prevalent dialysis population has reached 300,000 and in the USA 400,000, narrowing the gap between the two countries despite the major population differences. The longer survival of the general and dialysis populations in Japan has led to a rapidly growing prevalent population, which is now 75% the size of the treated US dialysis population.

Accompanying this growth is the substantial cost of treatment and its rate of growth over time. Since 1998–1999 the annual percent total growth in ESRD expenditure in the USA has averaged 8%, substantially higher than the overall inflation rate and higher than the overall Medicare general population expenditure growth rate (USRDS 2011 ADR, chapter 11, figure 11.4). The 8% growth is double the growth rate of the total population under treatment. Per person per year costs have increased 4–5% per year, which is mostly attributable to the cost of injectable medication and hospitalization due to infectious complication (USRDS 2011 ADR, chapter 11, figure 11.7). These realities led the US Congress to require Medicare to implement a new payment system which removes incentives for overprescribing medications, Quality Improvement Programs (QIPs) to address underutilization of services which may have an adverse impact on patient outcomes (Medicare Improvements for Patients and Providers Act of

2008 – MIPPA) and a rebasing of the payments to encourage the use of alternative home dialysis modalities. The new payment system fully bundles all dialysis services including intravenous (IV) medications such as ESAs, IV vitamin D, IV iron, IV carnitine and dialysis-related IV antibiotics, averaging the payments over peritoneal dialysis (PD) and hemodialysis (HD) populations. The PD population uses fewer injectable medications and has lower outpatient costs when compared to similar HD patients (USRDS 2011 ADR, chapter 11). The lower costs for PD create a financial incentive to use the home dialysis therapies in appropriate patients since the margins between payments and costs are greater in the PD verses the HD population. The new payment system was implemented January 1, 2011, and major changes have occurred in the use of dialysis modalities and reductions in the use of expensive medications.

Japan is facing similar realities, yet the vast majority of dialysis patients in Japan are treated with HD, a therapy which requires overhead costs for building dialysis centers, and investments in equipment with staffing by technicians, nurses, physicians and administrative personnel. Home dialysis therapies require less capital expenditures since the therapies are usually done by the patients or assistants in their own home setting. In the case of PD, the equipment costs are substantially lower than the cost of a HD machine. Newer equipment for daily home HD is also less expensive and less complicated, thereby making this therapy an alternative in appropriate candidates. In this series of articles on home dialysis therapies in Japan, the authors review the utilization of various home dialysis modalities and their experience with these therapies, providing a perspective on their applicability in Japan. These data will provide a perspective on alternative therapies that may be useful in Japan, which may inform medical practice and healthcare policy on the ESRD program and how it could change over time.

Allan J. Collins, MD, FACP
Professor of Medicine, University of Minnesota
Director, Chronic Disease Research Group
914 S. Eighth St
Suite S406
Minneapolis, MN 55404 (USA)
Tel. +1 612 347 5811, E-Mail acollins@cdrg.org

Suzuki H (ed): Home Dialysis in Japan.
Contrib Nephrol. Basel, Karger, 2012, vol 177, pp 3–12

A Kinetic Model for Peritoneal Dialysis and Its Application for Complementary Dialysis Therapy

Akihiro C. Yamashita

Department of Human Environmental Sciences, School of Engineering, Shonan Institute of Technology, Tsujido-Nishikaigan, Fujisawa, Kanagawa, Japan

Abstract

Kinetic models have been used in both hemodialysis (HD) and peritoneal dialysis (PD) therapies. Since many different theoretical models are available, users should choose one of these models along with the purpose of their studies. In general, simple models are useful for clinical investigations as well as clinical research, while rigorous models may be useful for engineers and cannot be utilized without an aid of computers. Several pieces of commercial software that include rigorous models are available for evaluation of peritoneal permeabilities as well as for constructing prescriptions. One of these pieces was clinically evaluated and high correlations with correlation coefficients >0.98 were found between clinical and recalculated values of total Kt/V for urea, total creatinine clearances and the ultrafiltration volume. Although the overall mass transfer-area coefficients (MTAC) of the peritoneal membrane is a diffusive parameter, it may become a useful tool for predicting peritoneal ultrafiltration by defining an index for peritoneal diffusive selectivity, the ratio of MTAC for urea to that for creatinine. It is recommended to use super high-flux dialyzers in PD+HD (complementary) combined therapy because it is the opportunity in a week to remove much middle and/or large molecules greater than β_2-microglobulin. Kinetic models are especially useful in treatments with relatively complex prescriptions such as PD+HD combined therapy, and may be a key to the further success of these modalities performed at home.

There are several modalities available for treating end-stage renal disease patients. Each patient is required to choose one of these modalities after understanding features of each treatment. Peritoneal dialysis (PD) is used to be known as the first choice of the treatment because it was believed that PD could preserve the residual renal function (RRF) longer than hemodialysis

(HD). However, since the choice of so-called super high-flux dialyzers that has high hydraulic permeability and high solute permeability as well as high biocompatibility [1] has become a standard with the use of ultrapure dialysis fluid [2], no significant difference has been reported in terms of preservation of RRF [3, 4]. Studies showed that local inflammation may greatly influence the preservation of RRF [5, 6]. There were so many factors that may directly or indirectly induce the local inflammation in classic HD treatment such as bioincompatibility of the dialysis membrane, water quality of dialysis fluid, etc.; however, most of these problems have already been solved in modern HD treatment. On the contrary, bioincompatibility of the dialysate for PD, including low pH, high glucose concentration and the existence of glucose degradation products, still remains a problem. Then there is the choice of PD as the initiation is becoming controversial for the purpose of preserving RRF.

Under such circumstances the choice of another modality is becoming more and more popular these days in Japan, that is, PD+HD combined therapy, also known as complementary dialysis recommended by an ad-hoc committee of the International Society for Peritoneal Dialysis (ISPD) in 2005. Although this modality is just a combination of PD and HD, the prescription may be even much more complicated than that for PD or for HD. This paper discusses a peritoneal transport model for PD and its application for complementary dialysis for the clinical use of prescription. How the kinetic model should be applied is also discussed for the further success of PD and PD-related modalities that are basically performed at home.

Theoretical

The first peritoneal transport model for PD was proposed by Henderson and Nolph [7], assuming only the diffusion would occur from the body compartment to the dialysate. Under such circumstances, the rate of mass transfer across the peritoneal membrane $\dot{m}$ [mg/min] may be written in the following form:

$$\dot{m} = PA(C_B - C_D) \tag{1}$$

where P is the peritoneal permeability [cm/min] and A is the effective surface area [cm^2] of the peritoneal membrane, C_B and C_D are the concentrations in blood and dialysate (mg/ml), respectively. In this model, a uniform structure of the peritoneal membrane as well as no stagnant layer adjacent to it was taken into account. Considering these effects, P should be replaced by the overall mass transfer coefficient K_o and equation 1 becomes:

$$\dot{m} = K_o A(C_B - C_D) \tag{2}$$

where the product of K_o and A is called the overall mass transfer-area coefficient (MTAC) [ml/min]. Babb et al. [8] and later Garred et al. [9] modified equation 2 by introducing convective mass transfer for small solutes from the blood to dialysate as follows:

$$\dot{m} = K_o\, A(C_B - C_D) + Q_u\, C_B \tag{3}$$

where Q_u is the ultrafiltration rate across the peritoneum [ml/min]. Another modification was made by Yamashita and Hamada [10], considering comprehensive convection between the blood and dialysate compartment as follows:

$$\dot{m} = K_o\, A(C_B - C_D) + Q_u \left(\frac{C_B - C_D}{2} \right) \tag{4}$$

Popovich et al. [11] introduced a more rigorous model based on the irreversible thermodynamic theory as follows:

$$\dot{m} = K_o\, A(C_B - C_D) + Q_u\, (1 - \sigma)\bar{C} \tag{5}$$

$$\bar{C} = C_B - f(C_B - C_D) \tag{6}$$

$$f = \frac{1}{\beta} - \frac{1}{\exp(\beta) - 1} \tag{7}$$

$$\beta = \frac{Q_u \cdot (1 - \sigma)}{K_o A} \tag{8}$$

$$Q_u = a_1 \exp(a_2 \cdot t) + a_3 \tag{9}$$

where $\bar{C}$ is an average concentration defined by equation 6, f is a weight function defined by equation 7, β is the Peclet number [–], σ is the Staverman's reflection coefficient [–], a_1 [ml/min], a_2 [min^{-1}], and a_3 [ml/min] are empirical ultrafiltration parameters. Equation 5 is the well-known Kedem-Katchalsky equation.

Rippe [12] proposed a new model in which the mass transfer resistances mostly exist at the blood vessels and assumed the existence of three kinds of pores that were different in sizes. These pores were termed the large pore (pore radius $r_p = 250$ Å), small pore ($r_p = 50$ Å), and ultra-small pore ($r_p = 4$ Å), respectively. The large pore is the only route for protein molecules to penetrate across the blood vessel. The small pore is responsible for small and middle molecule transport as well as about 50% of water transport. The ultra-small pore allows only water molecules to pass across, mimicking aquaporin-1 molecule that functions as mentioned above. They started from the same Kedem-Katchalsky equation and ended up with the following form for each pore:

$$\dot{m} = Q_u \cdot (1 - \sigma) \, \frac{C_B - C_D \cdot \exp(-\beta)}{1 - \exp(-\beta)} \tag{10}$$

Simplified models (equations 1–4) are useful as a clinician's tool and are often used to calculate MTAC values for small solutes such as urea and creatinine. Rigorous models (equations 5 and 10) can never be applied without the aid of a computer, which may be useful as an engineer's tool and may be available in the form of commercial software. The choice of model is therefore important for users before starting the studies, otherwise users would meet many different numbers of MTAC from the same clinical data because values are thoroughly dependent on the equations as well as the algorithm of the calculation.

Commercial Software for Peritoneal Dialysis

There are several pieces of commercial software for analyzing and prescribing PD therapy developed and available from PD solution companies. PD-Adequest® (Baxter Healthcare Co., Chicago, Ill., USA) has the longest history since 1986. PDC™, the first software based on the three-pore model was once distributed by Gambro Co. (Stockholm, Sweden) [13]. PatientOnLine™ is another choice (Fresenius Medical Care Co., Badhonburg, Germany) that is based on the peritoneal function test [14].

There are two other pieces from JMS Co. (Tokyo, Japan), PD-NAVI® for CAPD/APD and PHD-NAVI exclusively designed for PD+HD combined (complementary) therapy. PD-NAVI® includes two rigorous models, Popovich's model and the three-pore model, and employed a mathematically sophisticated curve-fitting technique to obtain unknown peritoneal transport parameters [15].

Clinical Applications of Kinetic Models
PD-NAVI® was demonstrated to show its clinical relevance. For this purpose, 83 CAPD/APD patients were selected from 32 local Japanese hospitals. Criteria for patient selection were as follows: (a) currently treated by CAPD or APD with V_D = 2,000 ml/exchange; (b) V_{urine} <500 ml/day, and (c) not combined with any other treatment. Clinical data were then taken based on the original PD-NAVI® protocol.

Figure 1 shows correlations between measured and recalculated total Kt/V for urea (Kt/V, left) and weekly total creatinine clearance (Ccr, right) in PD-NAVI®. Nice linear correlations between measured and recalculated values were found with correlation coefficients $r = 0.985$ and 0.994 respectively for Kt/V and Ccr. The similar results were observed for ultrafiltration with $r = 0.993$ (data not shown). PD-NAVI® was then shown to return reliable results at least when recalculation was made for clinical results.

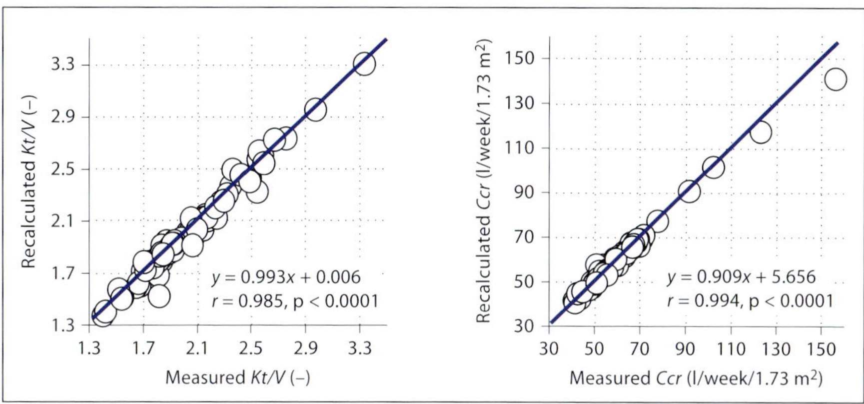

Fig. 1. Correlation between measured and calculated total *Kt/V* (left) and creatinine clearance (*Ccr*) (right).

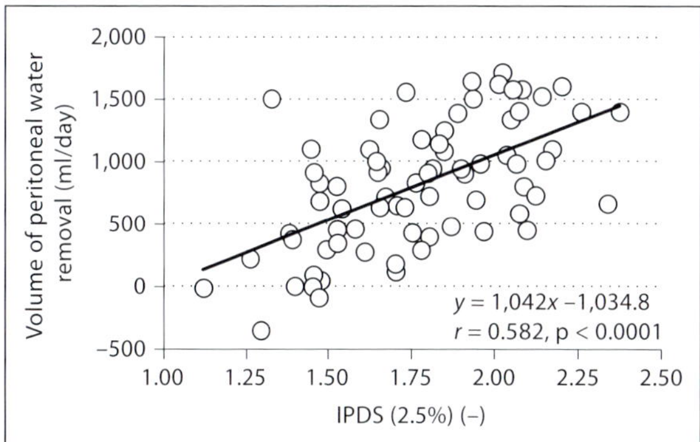

Fig. 2. Relationship between total volume of peritoneal water removal in a day and IPDS.

Since urea penetrates across the peritoneal membrane more quickly than creatinine, MTAC for urea will usually be larger than that for creatinine. We then defined the following parameter and termed it as the index for peritoneal diffusive selectivity (IPDS), i.e.:

$$IPDS = \frac{MTAC \text{ for urea}}{MTAC \text{ for creatinine}} \tag{11}$$

IPDS is usually much greater than unity, however when the peritoneal permeability becomes larger, IPDS would be approaching unity at which there is no difference in diffusive transport of urea and creatinine. Therefore, IPDS should correlate with the amount of ultrafiltration. The fact was demonstrated in figure 2 that shows a relationship between the total volume of peritoneal

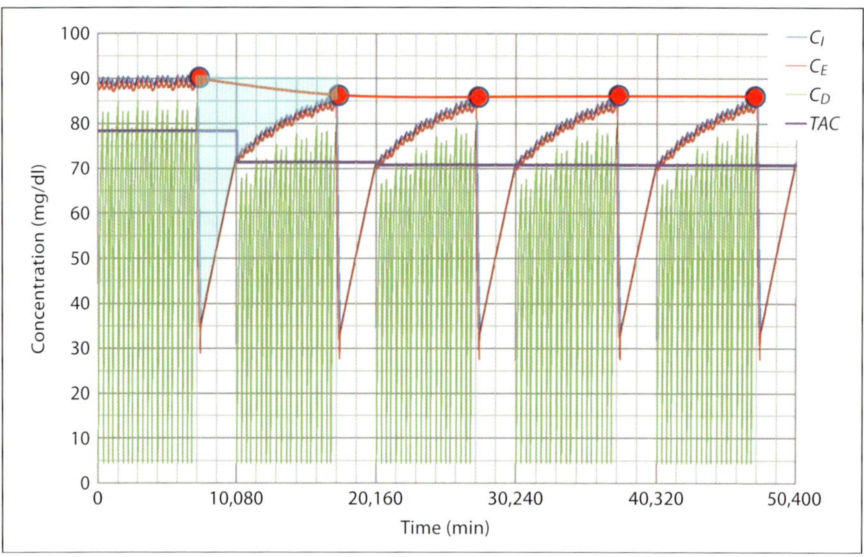

Fig. 3. Time courses of UN concentration profile in PD+HD combined therapy. C_I = Concentration intracellularly, C_E = concentration extracellularly, C_D = concentration in dialysate, *TAC* = time-averaged concentration.

water removal and IPDS. Another good linear correlation verified that although MTAC is just a diffusive parameter, IPDS may be a useful clinical predictor as well as a good evaluation tool of ultrafiltration.

PD and HD Combined (Complementary) Treatment

A modeled treatment schedule includes 5-day CAPD (4 exchanges/day) followed by one 4-hour HD and a 44-hour long no treatment period, and the calculation was made by Popovich's peritoneal transport model (equations 5–9) and the two-compartment model shown in the appendix (equations 10–18).

Figure 3 shows the time courses of urea-nitrogen (UN) concentration in PD+HD combined therapy for a modeled patient with a height of 165 cm and weight of 60 kg. Since urea is a small molecule and has little mass transfer resistance across the cellular membrane, the concentrations for UN in intra- and extracellular compartments are always almost the same and can be regarded as a constant for the first 5 days because the patient is on regular CAPD during this period of time. However, they rapidly decrease from 90 to 30 mg/dl by being treated with 4-hour HD and they increase abruptly with the 44-hour long no treatment time. Moreover, these concentrations increase even after PD is restarted with relatively lower rates. Therefore, once PD+HD combined

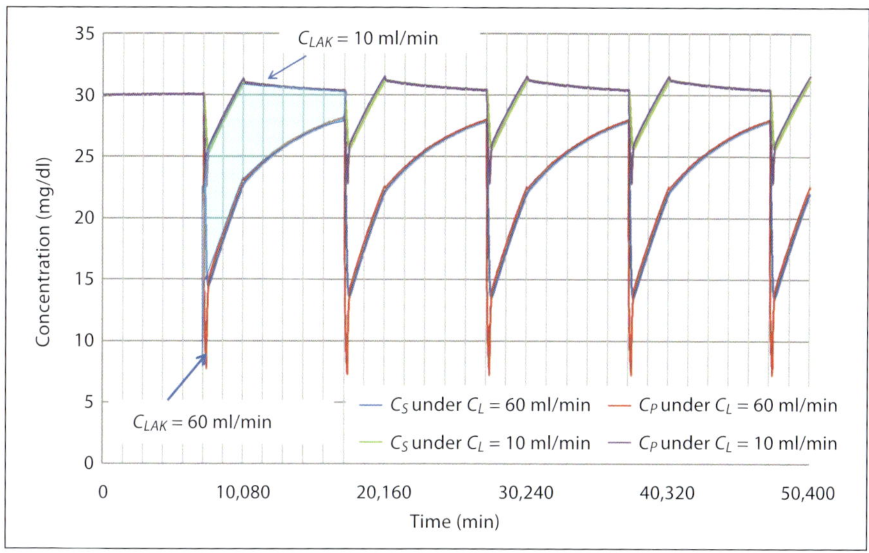

Fig. 4. Comparison of β_2-MG concentration in PD+HD combined therapy under C_{LAK} = 10 ml/min and C_{LAK} = 60 ml/min. C_S = Concentration interstitially, C_P = concentration in plasma.

therapy is started, concentrations never become constant even during the 5-day PD period.

If one defines the so-called 'pre-dialysis concentration' in this treatment as the concentration right before HD starts (shown as dots in figure 3), an decrease of only 5% may be expected. Moreover, this result is not drastically affected by the brand of dialyzer because most dialyzers have almost the same performances in terms of removing small solutes. What is good about this therapy, however, may be how low and how long the concentrations can be kept, then the area of the screened portion could be a key for evaluating the treatment. As a result, the time-averaged concentration (TAC) should decrease from 90 to 70 mg/dl, the reduction rate of which is approximately 22%, within 3 weeks after introducing PD+HD combined therapy.

The time courses of β_2-microglobulin (β_2-MG) concentration are shown in figure 4 with two different dialyzer clearances of 10 ml/min (low flux) and 60 ml/min (Japanese standard super high-flux under Q_B = 200 ml/min) for β_2-MG. Although the 'pre-dialysis concentration' would not change even when HD is done with a low-flux dialyzer, β_2-MG concentration may be beyond the original concentration of 30 mg/dl within a day or two after HD, unlike small solutes such as UN, since β_2-MG removal is strongly dependent on the brand of dialyzer. Therefore, it may be recommended to use a super high-flux dialyzer for removing β_2-MG or even larger molecules in PD+HD combined therapy because it is difficult to remove these large solutes with standard CAPD.

These results are clinically verified using the concept of 'clear space'. According to this concept, diminished RRF may be compensated for by one HD treatment for removing UN and β_2-MG with the use of super high-flux dialyzers in HD. Therefore, we concluded that performing HD once a week is equally matched to the RRF (residual urine volume of 640 ml/day) as far as removing urea and β_2-MG removal is concerned.

Conclusions

Historically speaking, a number of peritoneal transport models have been proposed both for clinical use and for a rigorous engineering tool, the latter is available in the form of commercial software. Clinically acceptable correlations were found between measured and recalculated values in total *Kt/V*, *Ccr*, and fluid removal by a commercial software (PD-NAVI®) that includes a rigorous peritoneal transport theory. Since a ratio of MTAC for urea to that for creatinine (IPDS) showed a linear correlation to the peritoneal water shift, it may become a useful predictor for fluid removal. Even a complex treatment (PD+HD combined therapy) may be well explained by the kinetic model that includes both the peritoneal transport model and a classic compartment model. Results may be useful for prescribing these modalities of treatment that are going to be performed at home.

References

1 Yamashita AC: Mass transfer mechanisms in high-performance membrane dialyzers; in High-Performance Membrane Dialyzers. Contrib Nephrol. Basel, Karger, 2011, vol 173, pp 95–102.
2 ISO: ISO/FDIS 1163: Quality of dialysis fluid for haemodialysis and related therapies.
3 McKane W, Chandna SM, Tattersall JE, Greenwood RN, Farrington K: Identical decline of residual renal function in high-flux biocompatible hemodialysis and CAPD. Kidney Int 2002;61:256–265.
4 Yamashita AC, Kotoku N: Does intermittent treatment decrease the residual renal function in shorter period of time? (In Japanese). J Jpn Soc Dial Ther 2007;40:464–466
5 Pecoits-Filho R, Heimburger O, Barany P, Suliman M, Fehrman-Ekholm I, Lindholm B, Stenvinkel P: Associations between circulating inflammatory markers and residual renal function in CRF patients. Am J Kidney Dis 2003;41:1212–1218.
6 Panichi V, Migliori M, De Pietro S, Taccola D, Bianchi AM, Norpoth M, Metelli MR, Giovannini L, Tetta C, Palla R: C Reactive protein in patients with chronic renal diseases. Ren Fail 2001;23:551–562.
7 Henderson LW, Nolph KD: Altered permeability of the peritoneal membrane after using hypertonic peritoneal dialysis fluid. J Clin Invest 1969;48:992–1000.
8 Babb AL, Johansen PJ, Strand MJ, Teckhoff H, Scriber BH: Bi-directional permeability of the human peritoneum to middle molecules. Proc Eur Dial Transplant Assoc 1973;10:247–262.

9   Garred LJ, Canaud B, Farrell PC: A simple kinetic model for assessing peritoneal dialysis. ASAIO J 1983;6:131–137.

10 Yamashita AC, Hamada H: A new simple kinetic model considering comprehensive ultrafiltration (in Japanese). J Jap Soc Dial Ther 1998;31:183–189.

11 Popovich RP, Pyle WK, Bomer JB, Moncrief JW: Peritoneal dialysis. Chronic replacement of kidney function. Am Inst Chem Eng Symp Series 187 1979;75:31–45.

12 Rippe B: A three-pore model of peritoneal transport. Perit Dial Int 1993;13(suppl 2):S35–S38.

13 Haraldsson B: Assessing the peritoneal capacities of individual patients. Kidney Int 1995;47:1187–1198.

14 Gotch FA, Lipps BJ, Pack PD: A urea kinetic modeling computer program for peritoneal dialysis. VIth International Course on Peritoneal Dialysis. Perit Dial Int 1997;17(suppl 2):347–351.

15 Hamada H, Sakiyama R, Yamashita AC, Okamoto M, Tojo KJ, Kumano K, Sakai T: Validation of a new analytical model for peritoneal transport model using rabbit in vivo experimental data. Nephrology 2000;5:59–64.

16 Hume R, Weyers E: Relationship between total body water and surface area in normal and obese subjects. J Clin Pathol 1971;24:234–238.

17 Yamashita A, Yoshimoto T, Ando K, Yoshimoto K, Hidai H, Sakai T, Sakai K: Estimation of cellular membrane clearance and fluid volume ratio intra- and extracellularly (in Japanese). Jpn J Artif Organs 1983;12:425–428.

Appendix

A classic two-compartment model was used for the calculation of concentrations in a modeled patient. A set of simultaneous differential equations was solved by the fourth-order Runge-Kutta technique.

1. For small solutes (urea and creatinine):

$$\frac{d\,(V_I C_I)}{dt} = G_I - K_c\,(C_I - X_c\,C_E) \tag{12}$$

$$\frac{d\,(V_E C_E)}{dt} = G_E + K_c\,(C_I - X_c\,C_E) - C_L\,C_E \tag{13}$$

$$\frac{dV_I}{dt} = 0 \tag{14}$$

$$\frac{dV_E}{dt} = -\,(Q_F - Q_S) \tag{15}$$

where X_c is the distribution coefficient at equilibrium [–] that can usually be assumed to be unity for small solutes, Q_S is the rate of substitution fluid into the body [ml/min], and $G_E = 0$ is assumed. Applying measured C_L for HD portion of the treatment, G_I can be determined since it is the only unknown parameter.

2. For β_2-MG:

$$\frac{d\,(V_S C_S)}{dt} = G_S - K_w\,(C_S - X_w\,C_P) \tag{16}$$

$$\frac{d\,(V_P C_P)}{dt} = G_P + K_w\,(C_S - X_w\,C_P) - C_L\,C_P \tag{17}$$

$$\frac{dV_S}{dt} = -\frac{3}{4}\,(Q_F - Q_S) \tag{18}$$

$$\frac{dV_P}{dt} = -\frac{1}{4}\,(Q_F - Q_S) \tag{19}$$

where X_w is the distribution coefficient at equilibrium [–] that may not be but is assumed to be unity, and $G_S = 0$ is assumed. Applying measured C_L for HD portion of the treatment, G_P can be determined as it is the only unknown parameter.

In all cases, if the patient has the RRF,

$$C_L = C_{LR} + C_{LAK} \tag{20}$$

where C_{LR} is the residual renal clearance and C_{LAK} is that of artificial kidney (dialysis).

V = total body fluid volume [ml]

= $(0.194786\,HT + 0.296785\,BW - 14.012934) \times 10^3$ (for males) [16]

= $(0.344547\,HT + 0.183809\,BW - 35.270121) \times 10^3$ (for females) [16],

where HT is the height in cm, and BW is the body weight in kg;

G_X = solute generation rate in the compartment 'X' [mg/min]

= determined from HD portion of clinical measurements.

K_c = cellular wall clearance [ml/min] = $0.320\,V\,\exp(-0.02519\,MW)$,

where MW is the molecular weight of the solute of interest [17].

K_w = capillary wall clearance [ml/min] = 40 ml/min for β_2-MG

$C_X(t)$: solute concentrations in compartment 'X' [mg/ml]

$V_X(t)$: volumes of the compartment 'X' [ml]

Subscripts: *I*: intracellular compartment; *E*: extracellular compartment; *S*: interstitial compartment; *P*: plasma compartment.

Akihiro C. Yamashita, PhD
Department of Human Environmental Sciences
School of Engineering, Shonan Institute of Technology
1-1-25 Tsujido-Nishikaigan, Fujisawa, Kanagawa 251-8511 (Japan)
Tel./Fax +81 466 30 0234, E-Mail yama@la.shonan-it.ac.jp

     Yamashita

Suzuki H (ed): Home Dialysis in Japan.
Contrib Nephrol. Basel, Karger, 2012, vol 177, pp 13–23

How Automated Peritoneal Dialysis Is Applied and Maintained in Japan

Hidetomo Nakamoto

Department of General Internal Medicine, Saitama Medical University, Saitama, Japan

Abstract

According to a nationwide statistical survey in Japan, only 9,858 patients (3.3% of dialysis patients) were on maintenance peritoneal dialysis (PD) at the end of 2009. In this survey, 8,635 patients answered questions about the PD method, while 1,223 patients did not respond. In Japan, at the end of 2009, 5,143 patients (59.6%) on PD were treated with CAPD and 3,492 patients (40.4%) on PD were treated with automated PD (APD). It is well known that around 20% of Japanese PD patients choose to apply and maintain PD + HD combination therapy. The number of PD + HD patients (1,569) accounted for 20.7% of the PD-treated patients (7,591). In Japan, patients with fluid overloading preferably select PD + HD combination therapy with or without icodextrin use. Young patients select APD while patients on PD suffered from fluid overloading with high transporter membrane. What then are the factors that effect APD selection in Japan? The use of various forms of APD has increased considerably in the past few years. Important factors that contribute to APD selection are better adjustment of APD to the patient's lifestyle and the flexibility that APD offers to patients. In addition, patients with APD will be able to have good quality of life (QOL). Young patients on PD select APD because of good QOL. It is well known that almost all of children younger than 19 years with end-stage renal disease (ESRD) are undergoing APD. APD has a pivotal role in the management of pediatric patients with ESRD. Children on APD had a lower incidence of peritonitis compared with those with CAPD. The switch from CAPD to APD resulted in better ultrafiltration, less edema, lower mean arterial blood pressure, lower peritonitis rate and fewer hospital admissions. As in young patients, APD is also good method to select in elderly patients on PD. The need for the exchange to be performed by another person is increased in elderly and handicapped ESRD patients, however APD therapy is a good selection for them because of the smaller number of manipulations, resulting in a substantial reduction of help required. In the future, telemedicine systems with APD may be play an important role for young and elderly patients on PD.

In recent years, important advances have been made in the treatment of patients with end-stage renal disease (ESRD) [1]. ESRD patients and their physicians must consider many factors, e.g. age, sex, profession, quality and length of life, when choosing a treatment regimen. Because of the limited number of donor organs, most patients must undergo dialysis [2, 3]. The distribution of patients with ESRD among transplantation, hemodialysis (HD) and peritoneal dialysis (PD) therapy differs dramatically in Japan and other countries.

According to a nationwide statistical survey in Japan, the total number of dialysis patients in Japan at the end of 2009 was 290,661, as determined from the facility survey. The number of dialysis patients in Japan at the end of 2008 was 283,421, an increase of 7,240 patients (2.6%) from the end of 2008. [4]. On the contrary, according to the facility survey, the number of PD patients was 9,858 at the end of 2009, an increase of 558 patients from the 2008 survey (9,300 PD patients). Moreover, the number of non-PD + catheter patients was 437 and that of new patients who were started on PD in 2009 but introduced to other therapies in the same year was 196. The total number of these PD therapy-related patients was 633. These 633 patients were not classified as PD patients in the previous surveys. The sum of these 633 patients and the above-mentioned PD patients (i.e. the total number of PD therapy-related patients) was 10,491. At least 500 or more PD patients were increased because in this 2009 survey, non-member facilities that treated only PD patients were included in the survey although they were not included in the previous surveys. However, the ratio of PD patients is very small compared to other countries.

One reason for this great difference in the number of dialysis patients in Japan was due to the good outcome of HD in Japan. In 2003, a prospective, observational HD study across seven countries, The Dialysis Outcomes and Practice Patterns Study (DOPPS), was reported [5, 6]. The crude 1-year mortality rates were 6.6% in Japan, 15.6% in Europe, and 21.7% in the USA. This data clearly demonstrates the good outcome of Japanese HD patients compared to other Western countries. On the other hand, what is the trend of Japanese ESRD patients on PD? Outcomes among PD patients differ considerably between and within countries [7, 8]. One of the most concerning differences is the varying technical survival and patient survival across countries [9]. We have previously already clearly reported that the outcome of Japanese PD patients including technical survival and patient survival are extremely good compared to other countries [10].

Dialysis Trends in Japan – A Nationwide Statistical Survey

In a nationwide statistical survey of 4,196 dialysis facilities conducted in Japan at the end of 2009, 4,133 facilities (98.5%) responded. The number of patients undergoing dialysis at the end of 2009 was determined to be 290,661, an increase of 7,240 patients (2.6%) compared with that of 2008. The number of patients

PET	<0.5	0.5–0.64	0.65–0.80	0.81–1.00	PET All	Unknown	Total
CAPD	176	589	642	206	1,613	3,530	5,143
(%)	(59.3)	(58.1)	(59.9)	(54.9)	(58.5)	(59.8)	(59.4)
NIPD	78	272	275	133	758	1,580	2,338
(%)	(26.3)	(26.9)	(25.7)	(35.5)	(27.5)	(26.8)	(27.0)
CCPD	40	146	145	34	365	789	1,154
(%)	(13.5)	(14.4)	(13.5)	(9.1)	(13.2)	(13.4)	(13.3)
Total	297	1,012	1,071	375	2,755	5,899	8,654
	(100.0)	(100.0)	(100.0)	(100.0)	(100.0)	(100.0)	(100.0)

newly introduced to dialysis was 37,566, a decrease of 614 (–1.6%). The number of decreased patients was 27,646, an increase of 380 (–1.4%). From this survey the increased number of patients was 9,920.

The number of dialysis patients per million at the end of 2009 was 2,279.5. The crude death rate of dialysis patients from the end of 2008 to the end of 2009 was 9.6%. Primary renal diseases in patients who newly started chronic dialysis in Japan in 2003 had diabetes mellitus (DM; 44.5%), chronic glomerulonephritis (CGN; 21.9%), nephrosclerosis (8.5%), and polycystic kidney disease (PCK; 2.3%). In 1993, primary kidney diseases were CGN (41.4%), DM (29.9%), nephrosclerosis (10.7%) and PCK (2.3%). The increased incidence of ESRD in diabetes in Japan was similar to the data of the United States Renal Data System (USRDS) report where the rate of DM and CGN had completely changed within 10 years. The dialysis patient population in Japan has been getting older on an annual basis.

In 2009, the mean age of new patients introduced to dialysis was 67.3 years; the mean age of the entire dialysis patient population was 65.8 years. In 1993, the mean age in all patients who started chronic dialysis was 59.8 years. The mean age of the dialysis population during the past 10 years has increased by 0.6–0.7 years annually [4].

Trends of CAPD and APD in Japan

It is well known that APD is now the fastest growing PD modality, and in some programs the majority of PD patients are treated with APD (table 1). The use of various forms of APD has considerably increased in recent years, mainly because of technological improvements and better adjustment to various patient lifestyles. The trend towards increased utilization of APD has been reported by French registry data: a rise in the use of APD to 36% in 2005 from 23% in 1995 [11]. According to a nationwide survey in Japan in 2005, 33.4% of PD patients were treated with APD. As well as other countries, a rise in the use of APD to 40.4% in 2009 from 34.4% in 2005 has been observed in Japan.

According to a nationwide statistical survey in Japan, only 9,858 patients (3.3% of dialysis patients) are on maintenance PD at the end of 2009. In this survey, 8,635 patients answered questions about the method of PD, while 1,223 patients did not respond. At the end of 2009, 5,143 patients (59.6%) on PD in Japan were treated with CAPD and 3,492 patients (40.4%) on PD were treated with APD. About 40% of PD patients were on maintenance APD in Japan in 2009 (table 1).

APD methods are traditionally divided into continuous cycling peritoneal dialysis (CCPD) and nocturnal intermittent peritoneal dialysis (NIPD). According to the nationwide survey in Japan, 2,338 patients were divided into NIPD and 1,154 were divided into CCPD. Of the APD patients, 67.1% were on NIPD and 32.9% were on CCPD.

According to the International Society of Peritoneal Dialysis (ISPD), APD is widely recommended for the management of high transporters [12]. A nationwide survey in Japan reported the D/P creatinine of PD patients at the end of 2009. Average D/P creatinine in patients on PD is 0.65 ± 0.14. How much is the average D/P creatinine according to the methods? In patients on CAPD, average D/P creatinine is 0.65 ± 0.13 (means). In patients on APD, NIPD and CCPD, averages of D/P creatinine are 0.66 ± 0.15 and 0.64 ± 0.14, respectively. There are no significant differences of D/P creatinine among these three groups. In other words, D/P creatinine is the same. Table 1 shows the method of selection of PD patients in Japan.

PD + HD Combination Therapy and Icodextrin in Japan

According to the results of the patient survey at the end of 2009, the number of patients who responded that they were undergoing only PD (referred to as 'PD-only patients') was 6,022. Therefore, the total number of these and the number of PD + HD patients (1,569) was 7,591. The other 2,267 patients were divided into unknown patients. Among these 7,591 PD patients, 1,197 (15.8%) underwent HD once a week, 191 (2.5%) did so twice a week, and 53 (0.7%) did so 3 times a week. PD + HD patients (1,569) accounted for 20.7% of the PD-treated patients (7,591). In addition, according to a nationwide statistical survey in Japan, 51.6% of ESRD patients on PD use polyglucose dialysis solution, i.e. icodextrin (Extraneal). Half of ESRD patients on PD use icodextrin. This is extremely high compared to other countries.

In CCPD patients, the patient carries a glucose-based PD solution in the abdominal cavity throughout the day, but performs no exchanges and is not attached to a transfer set. At bedtime, the patient hooks up to an automated cycler that will change the dialysis solution in his abdomen three or more times

  Nakamoto

in the course of the night. In the morning, the patient, with the last dwell of glucose-based or icodextrin (Extraneal) remaining in the abdomen, disconnects from the cycler and is free to go about daily activities. In Japan, CCPD with icodextrin is called E-APD. E-APD is a good method for PD patients with a high and high-average transporter to achieve a good ultrafiltration volume. The E-APD method is widely selected by APD patients in Japan.

Comparison of APD and CAPD

Over the last decade there has been an increasing application that peritoneal membrane transport characteristics play a crucial role in determining the morbidity, mortality and management of PD patients [12–16]. Patients with high peritoneal permeability (PET: high transporters) have been shown to have a substantially increased risk of death and technique failure, in spite of their more rapid diffusive clearance of urea and creatinine [16–19]. This increased risk has been attributed at least partly to rapid clearance of the glucose-associated osmotic gradient across the peritoneal membrane leading to ultrafiltration failure and fluid overload [14, 15]. There is evidence that patients with symptomatic fluid retention are 3.7 times more likely to be high than low transporters [20]. Modeling studies suggest that ultrafiltration in high transporters should be maximized by prescription of short dwell therapies by using APD [12]. Consequently, the ISPD Ad Hoc Committee on Ultrafiltration Management in Peritoneal Dialysis strongly recommends APD for the treatment of high transporter with impaired net ultrafiltration [12].

APD is widely recommended for the management of high transporters by the ISPD, although there has been no adequate evidence to date comparing the outcomes of APD and CAPD [12]. One prospective, open-label, randomized, multicenter controlled trial of APD vs. CAPD in 25 prevalent PD patients who were high or high-average transporters observed no significant changes in net filtration and was not statistically powered to evaluate survival outcomes [21]. A subsequent meta-analysis of three randomized controlled trials of APD vs. CAPD involving 139 patients did not find any differences in patient or technique survival, but was inadequately powered to assess these outcomes and did not perform subgroup analysis in high transporters [22]. For the most important point of method selection in APD, there is evidence which method has the better effect on survival and technique survival rate in patients on PD. There are some new findings of APD about the good effect on survival and technique survival rate. Johnson et al. [23] reported from an Australian and New Zealand Database that APD treatment is associated with a significant survival advantage in high transporters compared with CAPD (HR 0.59, 95% CI 0.35–0.87). However, APD treatment is associated with inferior survival in low transporters (HR 2.19, 95% CI 1.02–4.70). Cnossen et al. [24] reported that patient survival was not significantly different between APD and CAPD, whereas the technique of survival appeared to be higher in APD patients. Sun et al. [25] reported from the US Renal Data System (USRSD) that technique and patient survival are similar with APD and CAPD. Younger Chinese patients on APD have better patient and technique survival than do those on CAPD. However, there is a strong possibility that this benefit may be confounded or accounted for by baseline differences between the APD and CAPD populations.

How to Apply and Maintain APD in Japan

According to a nationwide survey in Japan, peritoneal membrane transport status has no effect on APD selection (table 1). Why then do Japanese patients not necessarily select APD with a high permeability of peritoneal membrane?

It is well known that around 20% of Japanese PD patients choose to apply and maintain PD + HD combination therapy. The number of PD + HD patients (1,569) accounted for 20.7% of the PD-treated patients (7,591). In Japan, patients with fluid overloading preferably select PD + HD combination therapy with or without icodextrin use. Young patients select APD when patients on PD suffered from fluid overloading with a high transporter membrane.

What then are the factors that effect APD selection in Japan? The use of various forms of APD has increased considerably in the past few years. Important factors contributing to APD selection were better adjustment of APD to the patient's lifestyle and the flexibility that APD offers. In addition, from the point of quality of life (QOL), patients with APD will be able to have good QOL. Young patients on PD select APD because of good QOL. Almost all young patients under 19 years of age select APD because they have go to school. It is well known that almost all children younger than 19 years with ESRD are undergoing APD [26]. APD has a pivotal role in the management of pediatric patients with ESRD [27]. Children on APD had a lower incidence of peritonitis compared to those with CAPD [28]. The switch from CAPD to APD resulted in better ultrafiltration, less edema, lower mean arterial blood pressure, a lower peritonitis rate and fewer hospital admissions [29].

Over a 24-hour period, APD involves only one connection in the night and only one disconnection in the morning. CAPD involves four connections and four disconnections. The smaller number of manipulations required from the patient could result in a substantial reduction in the incidence of peritonitis. It is well known that APD has been associated with improved compliance, lower intraperitoneal pressure and a lower incidence of peritonitis. Increased intraperitoneal pressure can be a problem during the application of PD and may result in the occurrence of hernias and fluid leaks causing discomfort (pleuroperitoneal communication) for some patients on PD. Lower abdominal pressure improves some complications of PD, including hernia and pleuroperitoneal communication.

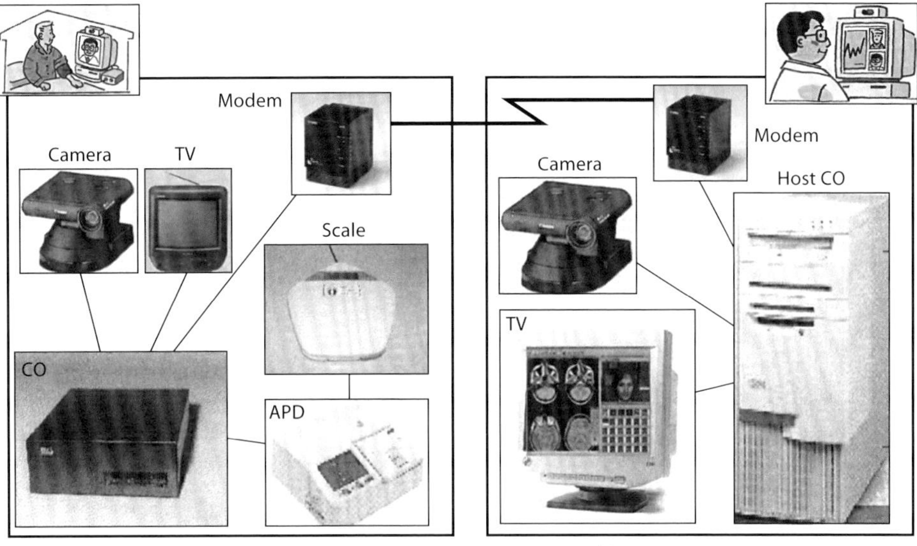

Fig. 1. Version 1.0 of a newly developed telemedicine system for CAPD patients using APD. In recent decades the rapid progression of information and telecommunication technology has evoked application of these techniques in the medical field. We have developed a telemedicine system to monitor elderly and handicapped PD patients by using an APD system (PD-mini; JMS Co., Tokyo, Japan).

As in young patients, APD is suitable in elderly patients on PD, especially in those with good residual renal function. The need for the exchange to be performed by another person is increased in elderly and handicapped ESRD patients [30]. APD therapy is a good selection for these patients because the smaller number of manipulations required results in a substantial reduction of help required. In fact, because of the increasing number of elderly patients on PD in Japan, these changes could explain the increased use of APD in general.

New Technology Using an APD Telemedicine System

For the purpose of monitoring elderly ESRD patients on PD, APD with a telemedicine system is a good selection for such cases. In recent decades, rapid progression of information and telecommunication technology has evoked application of these techniques in the medical field. We have developed a telemedicine system to monitor elderly and handicapped PD patients by using an APD system (PD-mini; JMS Co., Tokyo, Japan) (fig. 1) [31–34]. Using this system, we can retrieve all data directly, including blood pressure (BP), heart rate (HR), ultrafiltration volume (UF) and body weight (BW) (fig. 2).

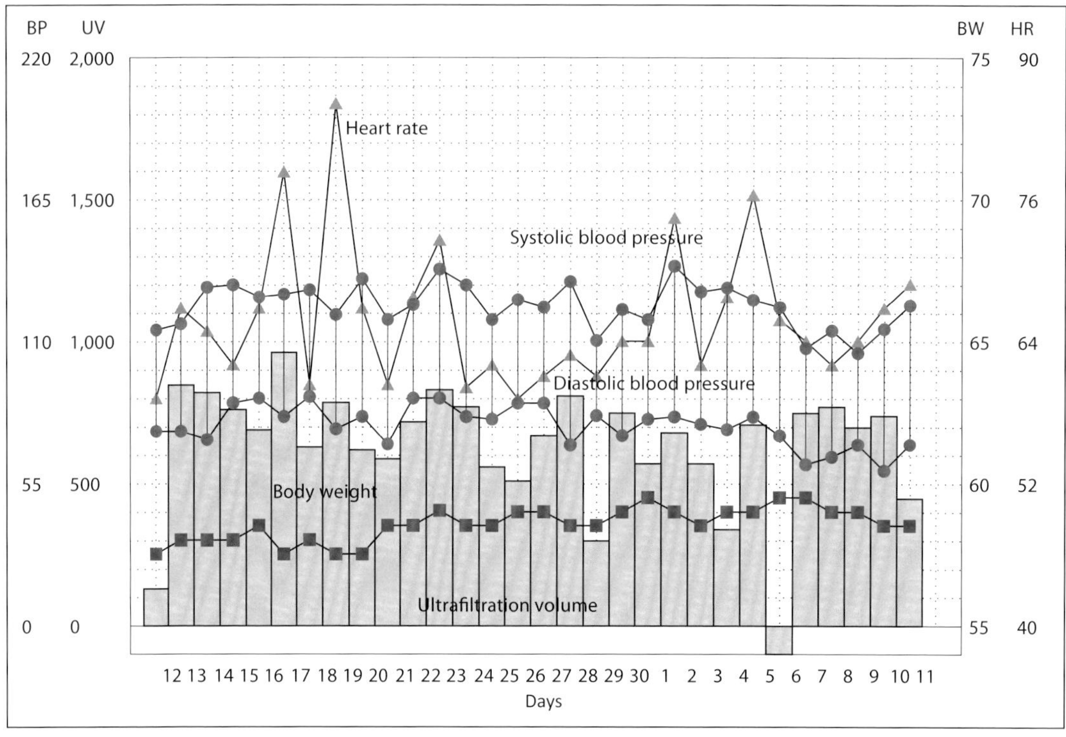

Fig. 2. Patient data on an internet website using the APD telemedicine system. With this system we can retrieve all data directly, including blood pressure (BP), heart rate (HR), ultrafiltration volume (UF) and body weight (BW).

This telemedicine system was constructed by two different systems including (i) a data transport system and (ii) a 'view send' system (video conference system). This system was constructed by two different systems including (i) a data-collecting and monitoring system by using APD and (ii) a medical record-sharing system in a computer internet website system by using an application service provider (ASP).

After 2003, to collect the data from a fully automatic device to a cellular phone, we developed a fully automatic data-collecting system named an I-converter (version 3.0; fig. 3). The data of PD patients including BP, HR, BW, blood glucose, and UF were directly sent to the main server constructed in a central data center by using an APD system and the I-converter. All data were collected on the central data center's main server which was directly connected to an internet website using application service provider technology (ASP). Doctors can check these data on an internet website anytime and anywhere with the patient's permission. This system has great advantages for elderly and handicapped patients because they do not need to visit the outpatient clinic. In addition, we can

                                                     Nakamoto

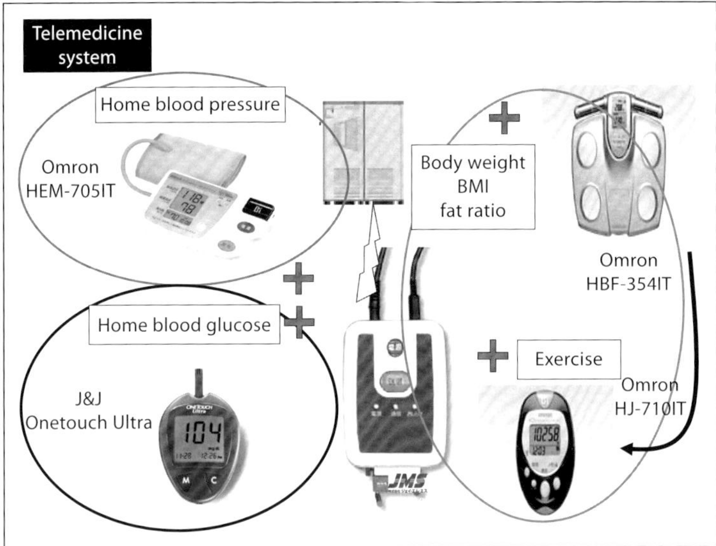

Fig. 3. Version 3.0 of telemedicine system to collect data at home.

monitor these patients at home in a real-time. In the future, telemedicine systems with APD may play an important role in young and elderly PD patients.

References

1 Blake PG, Bloembergen WE, Fenton SA: Changes in demographics and prescription of PD during the last decade. Am J Kidney Dis 1998;32(suppl 4):S44–S51.

2 Coles GA, Williams JD: What is the place of peritoneal dialysis in the integrated treatment of renal failure? Kidney Int 1998;54: 2234–2240.

3 Wolcott DL, Nissensson AR: Quality of life in chronic dialysis patients: a critical comparison of continuous ambulatory peritoneal dialysis and hemodialysis. Am J Kidney Dis 1988;11:402–412.

4 Japanese Society for Dialysis Therapy: An overview of regular dialysis treatment in Japan as of December 31, 2003 (in Japanese). Japan Society for Dialysis Therapy.

5 Young EW, Goodkin DA, Mapes DL, Port FK, Keen ML, Chen K, Maroni BL, Wolfe RA, Held PJ: The Dialysis Outcomes and Practice Patterns Study (DOPPS): an international hemodialysis study. Kidney Int 2000; 57(suppl 74):S74–S81.

6 Goodkin DA, Bragg-Gresham JL, Koenig KG, Wolfe RA, Akiba T, Angreucci VE, Saito A, Rayner HC, Kurokawa K, Port FK, Held PJ, Young EW: Association of comorbid conditions and mortality in hemodialysis patients in Europe, Japan, and the United States: the Dialysis Outcomes and Practice Patterns Study (DOPPS). J Am Soc Nephrol 2003;14:3270–3277.

7 Aloatti S, Manes M, Paternoster G, Gaiter AM, Molino A, Rosati C: Peritoneal dialysis compared with hemodialysis in the treatment of end-stage renal disease. J Nephrol 2000;13:331–342.

8   Davies SJ, Phillips L, Griffiths AM, Russell LH, Naish PF: What really happens to people on long-term peritoneal dialysis. Kidney Int 1998;54:2207–2217.

9   Blake PG: Trends in patient and technique survival in peritoneal dialysis and strategies: how are we doing and how we can do better? Adv Renal Replace Ther 2000;7:324–337.

10 Nakamoto H, Suzuki H, Kawaguchi Y: Why technique survival rate is so good in Japan? Perit Dial Int 2006;26:136–143.

11 European Renal Association (ERA) and European Dialysis and Transplant Association (EDTA) Registry: ERA-EDTA Registry Annual Reports 2006. Amsterdam, Academic Medical Center/Department of Medical Information, 2008. Available at www.era-edta-reg.org/files/annualreports/pdf/AnnRep2006.pdf (accessed November 2008).

12 Mujais S, Nolph K, Gokal R, et al: Evaluation and management of ultrafiltration problems in peritoneal dialysis. International Society for Peritoneal Dialysis Ad Hoc Committee on Ultrafiltration Management in Peritoneal Dialysis. Perit Dial Int 2000;20:S5–S21.

13 Rumpsfeld M, McDonald SP, Johnson DW: Higher peritoneal transport status is associated with higher mortality and technique failure in the Australian and New Zealand peritoneal dialysis patient populations. J Am Soc Nephrol 2006;17:271–278.

14 Davies SJ: Mitigating peritoneal membrane characteristics in modern peritoneal dialysis therapy. Kidney Int Suppl 2006;103:S76–S83.

15 Li PK, Chow KM: Maximizing the success of peritoneal dialysis in high transporters. Perit Dial Int 2007;27:S148–S152.

16 Brimble KS, Walker M, Margetts PJ, et al: Meta-analysis: peritoneal dialysis. J Am Soc Nephrol 2006;17:2591–2598.

17 Churchill DN, Thorpe KN, Nolph KD, et al: Increased peritoneal membrane transport is associated with decreased patient and technique survival for continuous peritoneal dialysis patients. The Canada-USA (CANUSA) Peritoneal Dialysis Study Group. J Am Soc Nephrol 2006;9:1285–1292.

18 Fried L: Higher membrane permeability predicts poorer patient survival. Perit Dial Int 1997;17:387–389.

19 Davies SJ, Phillips L, Russell GI: Peritoneal solute transport predicts survival on CAPD independently of residual renal function. Nephrol Dial Transplant 1998;13:962–968.

20 Tzamaloukas AH, Saddler MC: Murata GH: Symptomatic fluid retention in patients on continuous peritoneal dialysis. J Am Soc Nephrol 1995;6:198–206.

21 Bro S, Bjorner JB, Tofte Jensen P, et al: A prospective, randomized multicenter study comparing APD and CAPD treatment. Perit Dial Int 1999;19:526–533.

22 Rabindranath KS, Amato D, Vonesh E, et al: Automated vs. continuous ambulatory peritoneal dialysis: a systematic review of randomized controlled trials. Nephrol Dial Transplant 2007;22:2991–2998.

23 Johnson DW, Hawley CM, McDonald SP, Brown FG, Rosman JB, Bannister KM, Badve SV: Superior survival of high transporters treated with automated versus continuous ambulatory peritoneal dialysis. Nephrol Dial Transplant 2010;25:1973–1979.

24 Cnossen TT, Usvyat L, Kotanko P, van der Sande FM, Carter M, Leunissen KM, Levin NW: Comparison of outcomes on continuous ambulatory peritoneal dialysis versus automated peritoneal dialysis: results from a USA database. Perit Dial Int 2011;31:679–684.

25 Sun CY, Lee CC, Lin YY, Wu MS: In younger dialysis patients, automated peritoneal dialysis is associated with better long-term patient and technique survival than is continuous ambulatory peritoneal dialysis. Perit Dial Int 2011;31:301–307.

26 Oreopoulos D, Thodis E, Paraskevas KT: The promising future of long-term peritoneal dialysis. Int Urol Nephrol 2008;40:405–410.

27 United States Department of Health and Human Services, Public Health Service, National Institutes of Health, National Institute of Diabetes and Digestive and Kidney Diseases, Division of Kidney, Urologic, and Hematologic Diseases: USRDS 2007 annual data report. Atlas of end-stage renal disease in the United States. Bethesda, Unite States Renal Data System, 2007.

28 Fine RN, Ho M: The role of APD in the management of pediatric patients. A report of the North American Pediatric Renal Transplant Cooperative Study. Semin Dial 2002;15:427–429.

29 Fabian Velasco R, Lagunas Munoz J, Sanches Saavedra V, Men Brio Trejo GE, Qureshi AR, Garcia-Lopez E, et al: Automated peritoneal dialysis as the modality of choice: a single-center, 3-year experience with 458 children in Mexico. Pediatr Nephrol 2008;23:465–471.

30 Likopoulos V, Dombros N: Patient selection for automated peritoneal dialysis. Perit Dial Int 2009;29(suppl 2):S102–S107.

31 Nakamoto H, Hatta M, Tanaka A, Moriwaki K, Oohama K, Kagawa K, Wada H, Suzuki H: Telemedicine system for home automated peritoneal dialysis. Adv Perit Dial 2000;16: 191–194.

32 Nakamoto H, Kawamoto A, Tanabe Y, Nakagawa Y, Nishida E, Akiba T, Suzuki H: Telemedicine System for CAPD patients by using cellular phone. Adv Perit Dial 2003;19: 124–129.

33 Nakamoto H, Nishida E, Ryuzaki M, Sone M, Yoshimoto M, Itagaki K: Blood pressure monitoring system in patients on CAPD by using a cellular telephone. Adv Perit Dial 2004;40:105–110.

34 Nakamoto H: Telemedicine system in patients on CAPD. Perit Dial Int 2007; 27(suppl 2):S21–S26.

Hidetomo Nakamoto, MD
Department of General Internal Medicine, Saitama Medical University
38 Morohongo, Moroyama-machi, Iruma-gun
Saitama 350-0451 (Japan)
Tel. +81 1 492 76 1667, E-Mail nakamo_h@saitama-med.ac.jp

Suzuki H (ed): Home Dialysis in Japan.
Contrib Nephrol. Basel, Karger, 2012, vol 177, pp 24–29

Introduction and Maintenance Program for PD Based on PD Guidelines for Japan

Masaaki Nakayama

Fukushima Medical University School of Medicine, Department of Nephrology and Hypertension, Division of Dialysis Center, Fukushima, Japan

Abstract

Peritoneal dialysis (PD) guidelines for Japan were first published by the Japanese Society for Dialysis Treatment in 2009. They presented a concrete frame of PD practiced in Japan and stressed the timing of PD introduction as well as the clinical point of transfer to other modalities. The outlines of the guidelines and the issues to be addressed in the future are reviewed.
 Copyright © 2012 S. Karger AG, Basel

Recent Peritoneal Dialysis Trends and Frame of PD Guidelines in Japan

After nearly 30 years of peritoneal dialysis (PD) in Japan, there was a turning point of this modality in the mid-1990s. The rapidly increasing PD penetration until the early 1990s turned into a steady decline after this period (fig. 1). The emerging development of encapsulating peritoneal sclerosis (EPS) during the 1990s in Japan was thought to be the major reason for this decline. The degeneration of peritoneal membranes due to PD vintage was supposedly the primary reason for this development [1, 2] and it was suggested that exposure to bioincompatible PD solution was connected with the pathology [3, 4]. This facilitated the introduction in 2000 of biocompatible solutions (less glucose degradation products neutral solution) to be progressively used as standard solutions in Japan. Combination therapy with PD and HD was first performed in the mid-1990s in order to break away from bio-membrane peritoneum and enhance uremic control in patients who had lost residual renal function [5]. Nowadays, this unique PD method has become common practice and nearly 20% of PD patients in Japan are reportedly managed by combination therapy.

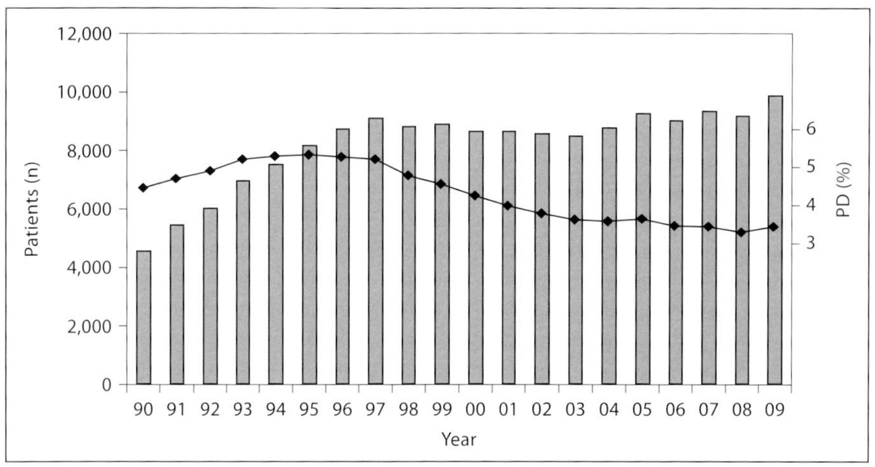

Fig. 1. PD population and PD utilization (%) among total dialysis patients in Japan (2000–2009).

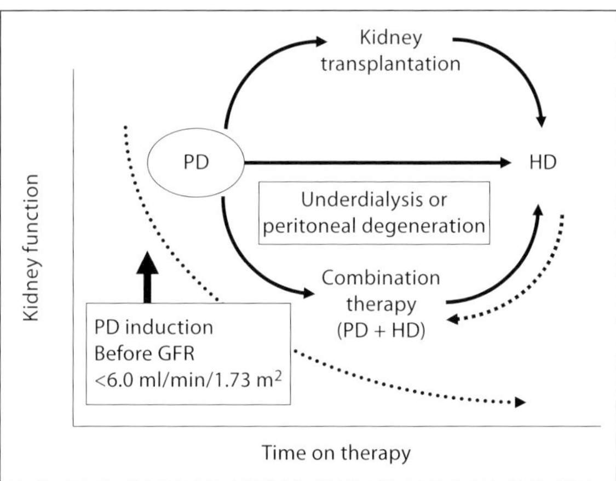

Fig. 2. Modern PD practice in the concept of strategic renal replacement therapy in Japan.

Due to the changing therapeutic situation described above, the Japanese Society for Dialysis Treatment published the first PD guidelines for Japan in 2009 [6]. When presenting a concrete frame of PD practiced in Japan (fig. 2), the three clinical points underlined in the guidelines were: (1) the guidelines promote PD as a standard initial treatment for integrated renal replacement therapy for end-stage renal disease, (2) they underline the significant role of combination therapy during the maintenance period, and (3) they recommend to stop PD if peritoneal degeneration progresses (table 1).

Table 1. Outline of the 2009 Japanese Society for Dialysis Therapy Guidelines for Peritoneal Dialysis (extracts from the guidelines)

Chapter 1: Initiation of peritoneal dialysis
1. Before the initiation of PD, sufficient information concerning hemodialysis, PD, and kidney transplantation should be provided to the patients, and the decision regarding modality choice must be made with the patient's consent (Evidence level VI: Committee opinion)
2. PD must be initiated concurrently with patient education to assure patients are adequately trained before starting self-treatment (Evidence level III)
3. Initiation of dialysis must be considered in patients with stage 5 CKD (GFR <15.0 ml/min/1.73 m^2 body surface area if they have signs or symptoms of uremia resistant to medical treatment (Evidence level VI: Committee opinion)
4. Initiation of dialysis is recommended before GFR reaches 6.0 ml/min/1.73 m^2 body surface area (Evidence level VI: Committee opinion)

Chapter 2: Adequacy of peritoneal dialysis
1. The adequacy of PD must be evaluated regularly according to the removal of accumulated waste products and state of hydration (Evidence level VI: Committee opinion)
2. The efficacy of PD is evaluated according to the weekly Kt/V urea, which should be maintained at a minimum target of 1.7, using a combined renal and peritoneal clearance of urea (Evidence level II)
3. To avoid fluid overload, an appropriate volume of ultrafiltration must be set, monitored and maintained (Evidence level III)
4. If signs and symptoms of uremia or malnutrition appear, despite the delivery of an adequate dialysis dose, changes in the prescription or therapy should be considered (Evidence level VI: Committee opinion)

Chapter 5: Discontinuation of peritoneal dialysis to avoid encapsulating peritoneal sclerosis
1. If progression of peritoneal deterioration is confirmed in patients with long-term PD or after peritonitis, discontinuation of PD should be evaluated with a due consideration of the risk of development of encapsulating peritoneal sclerosis (EPS) (Evidence level IV)
2. It is recommended to routinely perform the peritoneal equilibrium test (PET) to evaluate peritoneal deterioration (Evidence level VI: Committee opinion)

Background of PD Introduction at GFR not below 6.0 ml/min/1.73 m^2

In terms of PD induction, the guidelines recommend starting PD before the glomerular filtration rate (GFR) falls below 6.0 ml/min/1.73 m^2, even among asymptomatic patients [6]. Although the recommendation was opinion-based, it is quite pragmatic for several reasons. First, it is shown that the total dialysis dose (PD and residual renal function) positively impacts the outcome of incident PD patients, as shown in the CANUSA study [7]. Better survival was noted in subjects with weekly Kt/V urea levels >2.0 as well as weekly creatinine clearance (CCr) levels >60 liters. These values correspond to kidney function with a CCr of 8.0 ml/min/1.73 m^2 (equivalent to GFR 6 ml/min/1.73 m^2). Second, the recommendation considers the residual renal function being preserved after PD induction. Based on recent reports, including patients on biocompatible solution, it is estimated that the residual renal function declines at a speed of ca. 1.5 ml/min/1.73 m^2 per year [8–12]. Upon achieving adequate dialysis doses (weekly Kt/V urea 1.7, or CCr 55 liters) in cases on standard PD through 4 bag exchanges daily (weekly CCr 40 liters), it is roughly calculated that patients need a residual renal function >15–20 liters/week in CCr (GFR 2 ml/min/1.73 m^2) to undergo adequate PD. In these cases, PD therapy should be expected to continue for 3–5 years after achieving an adequate PD dialysis dose. The fact that most patients on combination therapy start within 3–5 years after PD induction may support this notion.

How to Access the Peritoneal Degeneration?

The term 'peritoneal degeneration' used in the guidelines is an abstract concept [6]. This embraces histological and functional changes of the peritoneum by function of PD vintage, which becomes a potential risk factor for developing EPS. Until now, no definite reliable tools or surrogate markers have been proven to predict EPS development exactly [13]. However, according to the reviews of the Japanese case reports on EPS, up to 75% of cases were reported to present a high transport membrane at EPS diagnosis [unpubl. data]. Also, there are reports to suggest the fact that progressive functional change by vintage of PD is closely related to the development of EPS thereafter [14–16]. Clinically, the peritoneal function test (peritoneal equilibrium test – PET) is simple and easy to perform on an outpatient clinic basis and does not need further specific equipment. With this background, the guidelines recommend to perform PET regularly and to standardize the monitoring of the appearance of peritoneal degeneration in clinical practice. Controversies remain on the issue of peritoneal function as a predictor for EPS [17, 18]. At present, an observational study on EPS development and its influencing factors is in progress in Japan, the NEXT-PD Study [19], which is expected to provide a novel insight into EPS in cases with less glucose degradation product neutral solution.

References

1   Nakayama M: The greater incidence of encapsulating peritoneal sclerosis is not the result of overdiagnosis. Perit Dial Int 2001; 21(suppl 3):S72–S74.

2   Kawanishi H, Kawaguchi Y, Fukui H, Hara S, Imada A, Kubo H, Kin M, Nakamoto M, Ohira S, Shoji T: Encapsulating peritoneal sclerosis in Japan: a prospective, controlled, multicenter study. Am J Kidney Dis 2004;44: 729–737.

3   Nakayama M, Kawaguchi Y, Yamada K, Hasegawa T, Takazoe K, Katoh N, Hayakawa H, Osaka N, Yamamoto H, Ogawa A, Kubo H, Shigematsu T, Sakai O, Horiuchi S: Immunohistochemical detection of advanced glycosylation end-products in the peritoneum and its possible pathophysiological role in CAPD. Kidney Int 1997;51:182–186.

4   Perl J, Nessim SJ, Bargman JM: The biocompatibility of neutral pH, low-GDP peritoneal dialysis solutions: benefit at bench, bedside, or both? Kidney Int 2011;79:814–824.

5   Fukui H, Hara S, Hashimoto Y, Horiuchi T, Ikezoe M, Itami N, Kawabe M, Kawanishi H, Kimura H, Nakamoto Y, Nakayama M, Ono M, Ota K, Shinoda T, Suga T, Ueda T, Fujishima M, Maeba T, Yamashita A, Yoshino Y, Watanabe S, PD+HD Combination Therapy Study Group: Review of combination of peritoneal dialysis and hemodialysis as a modality of treatment for end-stage renal disease. Ther Apher Dial 2004;8:56–61.

6   2009 Japanese Society for Dialysis Therapy Guidelines for Peritoneal Dialysis. Working Group Committee for Preparation of Guidelines for Peritoneal Dialysis, Japanese Society for Dialysis Therapy; Japanese Society for Dialysis Therapy. Ther Apher Dial 2010;14:489–504.

7   Churchill DN, Thorpe KE, Nolph KD, Keshaviah PR, Oreopoulos DG, Pagé D: Increased peritoneal membrane transport is associated with decreased patient and technique survival for continuous peritoneal dialysis patients. The Canada-USA (CANUSA) Peritoneal Dialysis Study Group. J Am Soc Nephrol 1998;9:1285–1292.

8   Fan SL, Pile T, Punzalan S, Raftery MJ, Yaqoob MM: Randomized controlled study of biocompatible peritoneal dialysis solutions: effect on residual renal function. Kidney Int 2008;73:200–206.

9   Szeto CC, Chow KM, Lam CW, Leung CB, Kwan BC, Chung KY, Law MC, Li PK: Clinical biocompatibility of a neutral peritoneal dialysis solution with minimal glucose-degradation products – a one-year randomized control trial. Nephrol Dial Transplant 2007;22:552–559.

10   Haag-Weber M, Krämer R, Haake R, Islam MS, Prischl F, Haug U, Nabut JL, Deppisch R, on behalf of the DIUREST Study Group: Low-GDP fluid (Gambrosol trio) attenuates decline of residual renal function in PD patients: a prospective randomized study. Nephrol Dial Transplant 2010;25:2288–2296.

11   Kim SG, Kim S, Hwang YH, Kim K, Oh JE, Chung W, Oh KH, Kim HJ, Ahn C, Korean Balnet Study Group: Could solutions low in glucose degradation products preserve residual renal function in incident peritoneal dialysis patients? A 1-year multicenter prospective randomized controlled trial (Balnet Study). Perit Dial Int 2008;28(suppl 3): S117–S122.

12   Jansen MA, Hart AA, Korevaar JC, Dekker FW, Boeschoten EW, Krediet RT, NECOSAD Study Group: Predictors of the rate of decline of residual renal function in incident dialysis patients. Kidney Int 2002;62:1046–1053.

13   Korte MR, Sampimon DE, Betjes MG, Krediet RT: Encapsulating peritoneal sclerosis: the state of affairs. Nat Rev Nephrol 2011; 7:528–538.

14   Nakayama M, Ikeda M, Katoh N, Hayakawa H, Numata M, Otsuka Y, Yamamoto R, Yamamoto H, Yokoyama K, Kubo H, Kawaguchi Y, Hosoya T: Long-standing high-transport membrane as a risk factor for EPS development after PD withdrawal: an analysis based on changes in peritoneal function during and after CAPD withdrawal (in Japanese). Nihon Jinzo Gakkai Shi 2002;44: 396–401.

15   Otsuka Y, Nakayama M, Ikeda M, Sherif AM, Yokoyama K, Yamamoto H, Kawaguchi Y: Restoration of peritoneal integrity after withdrawal of peritoneal dialysis: characteristic features of the patients at risk of encapsulating peritoneal sclerosis. Clin Exp Nephrol 2005;9:315–319.

16   Yamamoto R, Otsuka Y, Nakayama M, Maruyama Y, Katoh N, Ikeda M, Yamamoto H, Yokoyama K, Kawaguchi Y, Matsushima M: Risk factors for encapsulating peritoneal sclerosis in patients who have experienced peritoneal dialysis treatment. Clin Exp Nephrol 2005;9:148–152.

17 Balasubramaniam G, Brown EA, Davenport A, Cairns H, Cooper B, Fan SL, Farrington K, Gallagher H, Harnett P, Krausze S, Steddon S: The Pan-Thames EPS Study: treatment and outcomes of encapsulating peritoneal sclerosis. Nephrol Dial Transplant 2009;24:3209–3215.

18 Sampimon DE, Coester AM, Struijk DG, Krediet RT: The time course of peritoneal transport parameters in peritoneal dialysis patients who develop encapsulating peritoneal sclerosis. Nephrol Dial Transplant 2011; 26:291–298.

19 Kawanishi H, Nakayama M, Miyazaki M, Honda K, Tomo T, Kasai K, Nakamoto H, NEXT-PD Study Group: Prospective multi-center observational study of encapsulating peritoneal sclerosis with neutral dialysis solution – the NEXT-PD study. Adv Perit Dial 2010;26:71–74.

Masaaki Nakayama, MD
Fukushima Medical University School of Medicine
1 Hikarigaoka, Fukushima City
Fukushima 960-1295 (Japan)
Tel. +81 24 547 1206, E-Mail masanaka@fmu.ac.jp

Suzuki H (ed): Home Dialysis in Japan.
Contrib Nephrol. Basel, Karger, 2012, vol 177, pp 30–37

Appropriate Drug Dosing in Patients Receiving Peritoneal Dialysis

Sumio Hirata · Daisuke Kadowaki

Division of Clinical Pharmacology, Center for Clinical Pharmaceutical Sciences,
Faculty of Pharmaceutical Sciences, Kumamoto University, Kumamoto, Japan

Abstract

The quantity of drugs removed during peritoneal dialysis is substantially lower than that during hemodialysis, and thus, the supplemental administration of drugs, even when they are efficiently removed during hemodialysis, is not necessary in patients receiving continuous ambulatory peritoneal dialysis (CAPD). However, because CAPD is a continuous hemocatharsis procedure, the cumulative removal of renally excretable drugs is higher in CAPD patients than in hemodialysis patients between sessions. Therefore, the weekly dosage of a drug can be approximately the same in CAPD patients and hemodialysis patients, and dosing design for patients with a pre-end-stage renal disease in the period prior to the initiation of dialysis can be applied to CAPD patients. Nevertheless, an appropriate dosage regimen, based on drug clearance, should be determined, because drug clearance is enhanced in patients receiving automated peritoneal dialysis, compared with those receiving CAPD, and also in those with urine output, compared to anuric patients. In addition, when residual renal function is impaired in CAPD patients with urine output, the decreased drug clearance must be compensated for by introducing a weekly hemodialysis treatment in some cases. Thus, careful consideration should be exercised in cases where drugs that have adverse effects on renal function are being administered, such as drugs that exert nephrotoxic effects and cause renal ischemia in CAPD patients. In the case of CAPD-related peritonitis, when an antibiotic that binds strongly to a protein is intravenously injected, the drug concentration in the peritoneal dialysate is low because only the unbound drug can be transported to the peritoneal dialysate. For this reason, when drugs, such as teicoplanin, that bind strongly to a protein are administered to CAPD patients with peritonitis, an intraperitoneal route is preferable to an intravenous route.

Drug Clearance during CAPD

Drug clearance during CAPD is dependent on the drain volume. When a patient is on a regimen of 2-liter exchanges four times per day, the concentration of urea, a small molecule of 60 Da, in the dialysate becomes equal to that in the plasma within a few hours, resulting in a clearance rate of 8 liters/day (5.6 ml/min). With ultrafiltration attributed to glucose in the dialysate, the actual daily drain volume in this case would be approximately 9 liters during CAPD. In addition, because many CAPD patients have some residual renal function, clearance would be further increased and the magnitude of the clearance would be dependent on the urine output of the individual patient. However, CAPD patients produce near-isotonic urine, so the maximum clearance of urea is only around 7 ml/min (see below). Peritoneal clearance can be calculated using the following equation:

$$\text{Peritoneal urea clearance} = D/P \ / \ VD/t$$

Here, VD is the dialysate drain volume (ml), t is the dwell time (min), D is the drug concentration in the dialysate, and P is the plasma drug concentration. Since urea moves rapidly into the peritoneal dialysate, D becomes approximately equal to P, and the above equation can be expressed as:

$$\text{Peritoneal clearance (ml/min)} \approx VD/t$$

For example, when a CAPD patient produces 1 liter of urine per day, peritoneal urea clearance $\approx$2 liters $\times$ 4/day (dialysate volume) + 1 liter/day (ultrafiltration volume), urea clearance = peritoneal clearance for urea + 1 liter (urine output) = 10 liters/day $\approx$6.94 ml/min. While the D/P ratio of urea after a 6-hour dwell time is approximately 1, that of creatinine, which has a higher molecular weight (113 Da), is 0.7–0.8; therefore, creatinine clearance would be 4–6 ml/min in CAPD patients (fig. 1) [1, 2]. Even though CAPD is a continuous hemocatharsis method, it achieves considerably low levels of clearance, which are barely adequate for preventing uremia [3]. This means that CAPD is not an effective hemocatharsis approach for treating patients with acute drug intoxication, and its influence on short-term pharmacokinetics is nearly negligible [4].

The peritoneum is a natural high-performance membrane with a surface area that is approximately the same size as that of the body surface. The endothelial cells of the peritoneum contain capillaries with a pore size of 40–200 Å. Compared with hemodialysis membranes, larger molecules and proteins are able to pass through the peritoneal membrane, but it contains markedly fewer pores. Therefore, the area of the peritoneum used for filtering is approximately the same size as, or slightly larger than, that of the typical hemodialysis membrane. However, the peritoneum has a markedly lower solute transport capacity

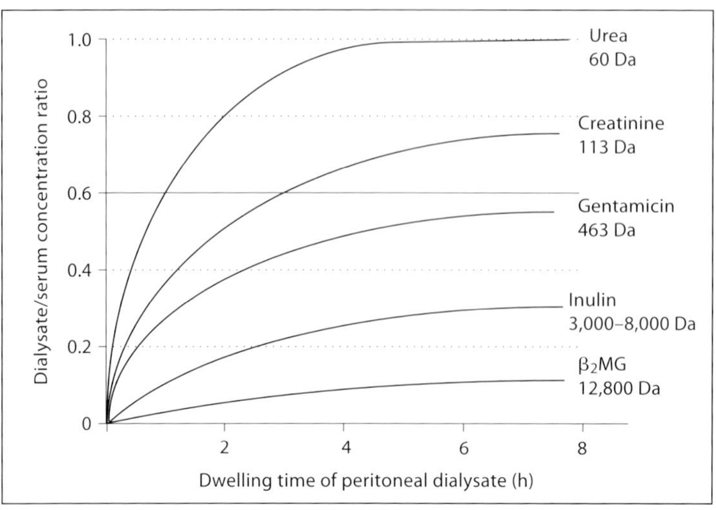

Fig. 1. Relationship between solute molecular weight, D/P ratio and clearance [1, 2]. D = Dialysate solute level; P = plasma solute level.

than the typical hemodialysis membrane for a given duration. This means that all drugs, without exception, should be removed preferentially during hemodialysis, rather than during CAPD. While urea and creatinine in dialysate plasma reach equilibrium relatively quickly, the concentration of inulin (3,000–8,000 Da) in the dialysate is roughly 30% of that in the plasma after an 8-hour dwell time, which indicates that the removal of medium-sized solutes continues during long dwell peritoneal dialysis [5].

Drug Regimen Design for CAPD Patients

Factors that determine drug dialyzability in CAPD patients include protein-binding, volume of distribution (V_d), molecular size, hydrophilicity (or liposolubility), peritoneal permeability and surface area, blood flow, dwell time, and dialysate glucose concentration [6]. Among these, a high V_d and a high protein binding rate are associated with low drug clearance during both hemodialysis and peritoneal dialysis.

As described earlier, drug clearance is extremely slow during CAPD, typically, a maximum clearance rate of 4–7 ml/min even for low molecular weight drugs. In most cases, the proportion of clearance by CAPD to total clearance is very small, so the same dosing regimen can be used in both CAPD patients and in patients with a pre-end-stage renal disease with a glomerular filtration rate of 5–10 ml/min. However, drugs with a low level of extrarenal clearance, a low protein binding rate, and/or a small V_d, such as aminoglycoside antibiotics,

Hirata · Kadowaki

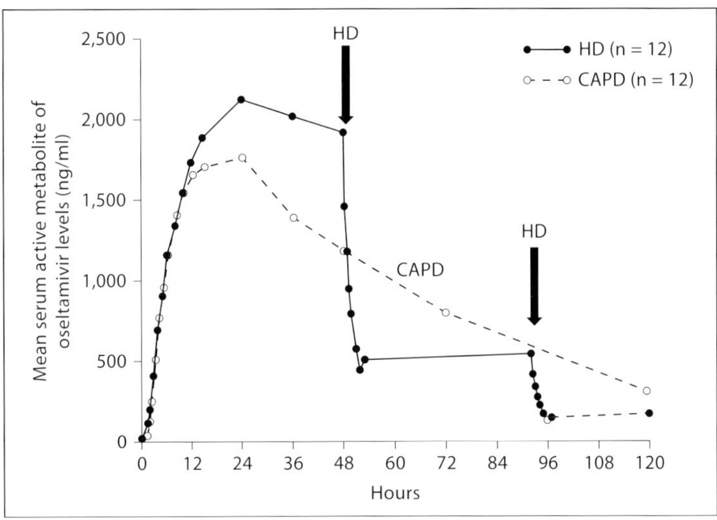

Fig. 2. Consecutive change in mean serum levels of active metabolite of oseltamivir in patients undergoing CAPD and HD [7].

β-lactam antibiotics, and the antiviral oseltamivir, are removed more completely in patients during CAPD than in hemodialysis patients between sessions. Ro 64-0802, which is the de-esterified active form of oseltamivir, has a low degree of protein binding (3%) and a small V_d (0.37 liter/kg), and is easily removed during both hemodialysis and CAPD. After a single dose of 75 mg of oseltamivir, rapid drug clearance occurs during hemodialysis, whereas during CAPD, drug clearance is gradual and continuous; when the IC90 for a viral strain is 100 ng/ml, an effective drug concentration can be retained for 5 days (fig. 2) [7]. Oseltamivir is an anti-influenza drug that is effective with a single dose in clinical cases undergoing both CAPD and hemodialysis. Nevertheless, depending on the drug type, a decrease in blood drug levels during CAPD must be taken into consideration when designing a dosage regimen.

Drug clearance for a given duration is markedly lower during CAPD than during hemodialysis. However, because it is a continuous procedure, weekly clearance is not largely different between CAPD patients and hemodialysis patients, provided that a reasonable urine output is maintained. When weekly drug clearance was compared with respect to molecular size, small molecules were preferentially removed to a greater extent during hemodialysis than during CAPD, while mid-sized and large molecules were removed more preferentially, if not similarly, during CAPD than during hemodialysis, depending on the type of the membrane being used. The difference between CAPD and hemodialysis is the most prominent with small molecules, such as urea and creatinine. However, only a few molecules, such as lithium carbonate and ethanol, are smaller than urea and

Table 1. PK-PD parameters and antibiotic dosing recommendation for HD, CAPD and APD patients [8]

	Cefazolin	Cefepim	Tobramycin	Vancomycin
PK-PD parameters				
Urinary excretion rate	85%	80%	80%	90%
Protein binding rate	80%	12%	Less than 5%	34–55%
Volume of distribution	0.22 L/kg	0.25 L/kg	0.28 L/kg	0.9–1.0 L/kg
Molecular weight	566.6 Da	571.5 Da	467.5 Da	1485.7 Da
PK-PD parameters which quantify the activity of an antibiotic	Time above MIC (time dependent)	Time above MIC (time dependent)	Cmax/MIC (concentration dependent)	AUC/MIC
Dosing recommendation				
Hemodialysis	500–1000 mg after HD	1000 mg after HD	5 mg/kg after HD	LD 20 mg/kg, MD 10 mg/kg after HD
CAPD Intermittent (once daily)	15 mg/kg	1 g	0.6 mg/kg	15–30 mg/kg every 5–7 days
CAPD Continuous (mg/L, all exchabges)	LD 500 mg/L, MD 125 mg/L IP	LD 500 mg/L, MD 125 mg/L IP	LD 8 mg/L, MD 4 mg/L IP	LD 1000 mg/L, MD 25 mg/L IP
APD Intermittent (mg/kg)	20 mg/kg IP once per day, in long day dwell	1 g IP one exchange per day	LD 1.5 mg/kg IP in long dwell, then 0.5 mg/kg IP each day in long day dwell	LD 30 mg/kg in long dwell, repeat dosing 15 mg/kg IP in long dwell every 3–5 days, following levels

PK-PD = Pharmacokinetics-pharmacodyamics; MIC = minimum inhibitory concentration; AUC = Area Under the serum concentration time Curve; Cmax = peak serum level; LD = loading dose, MD = maintenanc dose in mg; IP = intraperitoneal administration.
Residual renal function (defined as >100 mL/day urine output) should be empirically increased by 25%.

creatinine, and thus, it is not necessary to use a different total dose for CAPD and hemodialysis patients. Exceptions to this principle are regimens for drugs that are removed rapidly during hemodialysis. In this case, supplemental dosing is required in hemodialysis patients, but not in CAPD patients (table 1) [8].

It has been reported that a decrease in urine output results in a decrease in the renal clearance of urea, creatinine, and phosphorus, but this is compensated for by an enhanced peritoneal clearance [9]. However, when patients become anuric, uremia cannot be prevented solely by peritoneal clearance during CAPD, and once a week hemodialysis treatments are required in some CAPD cases. For CAPD patients with urine output, an overdose of the following drugs should be avoided to preserve residual renal function: non-steroidal anti-inflammatory drugs which induce renal ischemia; renin-angiotensin system inhibitors; contrast agents; diuretics; nephrotoxic aminoglycoside antibiotics; those which induce urinary tract obstructions, such as acyclovir, and those which increase levels of calcium-phosphate products such as concomitant use of calcium preparation and large dose of activated vitamin D [10, 11]. Regimens of these drugs for patients with residual renal function should be different from those for anuric patients. The administration of aminoglycoside antibiotics has not in the past been recommended for CAPD patients with urine output, but this restriction was recently removed [8] after several studies showed that these antibiotics had no adverse effects on residual renal function [12–14]. Furthermore, it was reported on the basis of the pharmacokinetic-pharmacodynamic theory that once-daily aminoglycoside administration results in higher antibiotic effects and reduces the duration of exposure of proximal tubule cells to the aminoglycoside, thereby resulting in a significantly lower incidence rate of nephropathy compared with a three-times-daily regimen [15]. This suggests that a once-daily intraperitoneal administration of an aminoglycoside would be appropriate for the treatment of peritonitis in CAPD patients, since it would be expected to cause less nephrotoxicity and ototoxicity than multiple-daily intraperitoneal administration [14]. Considering that the co-administration of an aminoglycoside and vancomycin, especially with multiple-daily aminoglycoside, tends to cause nephropathy [16], it is recommended to opt for a once-daily aminoglycoside administration when both antibiotics are required.

Intraperitoneal Dosing and Peritonitis in CAPD Patients

In general, intraperitoneal dosing in peritoneal dialysis patients (i.e. adding a drug to the dialysis bag) is currently restricted to antibiotics and heparin, although other substances, such as insulin, were administered via this route in the past. Drugs that are administered intraperitoneally move rapidly into the bloodstream [17] and have a high bioavailability (50–92%) [6]. Indeed, it was reported that intraperitoneal administration achieves therapeutic concentrations at a level similar to that for an intravenous injection and that the outcomes of antibiotic treatment are generally comparable between intraperitoneal and intravenous routes in patients with peritonitis [18]. Drugs that bind weakly to proteins, such as aminoglycoside antibiotics, move into the peritoneal cavity at high concentrations when administered intravenously, while the concentration of intraperitoneally administered drugs remain higher than blood concentrations; thus, these drugs are suitable for both intravenous and intraperitoneal administration [14].

On the other hand, antibiotics that bind strongly to protein (>90%), such as cefoperazone, ceftriaxone, and teicoplanin, move rapidly into the bloodstream after intraperitoneal administration, because proteins rarely persist within the peritoneal cavity, and thus a large fraction of unbound drug becomes available to move into the bloodstream [19]. Conversely, when administered intravenously, the availability of unbound forms of these antibiotics for moving into the peritoneal cavity is low in the bloodstream, and, as a result, they are not effective for treating peritonitis [20, 21].

Peritoneal permeability is increased in CAPD patients with peritonitis [22], thereby enhancing the transport of intraperitoneally administered drugs into the bloodstream. A previously recommended teicoplanin regimen for CAPD patients with peritonitis is as follows: an intravenous injection of 400 mg on the first day; intraperitoneal administration of 40 mg four times daily (addition of 40 mg teicoplanin to four 2-liter bags/day) during the first week; intraperitoneal administration of 40 mg twice daily 40 mg (addition of 40 mg teicoplanin to two 2-liter bags/day) during the second week, and a daily intraperitoneal administration of 40 mg (addition of 40 mg teicoplanin to one 2-liter bag/day) during the third week [23]. In addition, the administration of teicoplanin at 10 mg/kg body weight every 24 h has been proposed for treating infectious diseases other than peritonitis in CAPD patients [21]. The recommended intraperitoneal vancomycin dosing for anuric CAPD patients with peritonitis is an intraperitoneal administration of 15–30 mg/kg body weight every 5–7 days or a 1,000 mg/l loading dose at each exchange followed by a 25 mg/l maintenance dose at each exchange [8].

References

1 Paniagua R, Amato D, Vonesh E, Correa-Rotter R, Ramos A, Moran J, Mujais S, Mexican Nephrology Collaborative Study Group: Effects of increased peritoneal clearances on mortality rates in peritoneal dialysis: ADEMEX, a prospective, randomized, controlled trial. J Am Soc Nephrol 2002;13:1307–1320.

2 Brophy DF, Sowinski KM, Kraus MA, Moe SM, Klaunig JE, Mueller BA: Small and middle molecular weight solute clearance in nocturnal intermittent peritoneal dialysis. Perit Dial Int 1999;19:534–539.

3 Keller E, Reetze P, Schollmeyer P: Drug therapy in patients undergoing continuous ambulatory peritoneal dialysis. Clinical pharmacokinetic considerations. Clin Pharmacokinet 1990;18:104–117.

4 Venkataraman V, Nolph KD: Preservation of residual renal function – an important goal. Perit Dial Int 2000;20:392–395.

5 Popovich RP: Transport kinetics; in Norph KD (ed): Peritoneal Dialysis. Boston, Nijhoff, 1985, pp 1–155.

6 O'Brien MA, Mason NA: Systemic absorption of intraperitoneal antibiotics in continuous ambulatory peritoneal dialysis. Clin Pharm 1992;11:246–254.

7 Kokai Y, Suzuki M, Matsuzawa M, Takasugi M: Pharmacology and pharmacokinetics of oseltamivir phosphate, the oral anti-influenza virus agent (in Japanese). Kagaku Ryoho No Ryoiki 2001;17:103–111.

8 Piraino B, Bailie GR, Bernardini J, Boeschoten E, Gupta A, Holmes C, Kuijper EJ, Li PK, Lye WC, Mujais S, Paterson DL, Fontan MP, Ramos A, Schaefer F, Uttley L, ISPD Ad Hoc Advisory Committee: Peritoneal dialysis-related infections recommendations: 2005 update. Perit Dial Int 2005;25:107–131.

9   Bammens B, Evenepoel P, Verbeke K, Vanrenterghem Y: Time profiles of peritoneal and renal clearances of different uremic solutes in incident peritoneal dialysis patients. Am J Kidney Dis 2005;46:512–519.

10 Tzamaloukas AH, Raj DS, Onime A, Servilla KS, Vanderjagt DJ, Murata GH: The prescription of peritoneal dialysis. Semin Dial 2008;21:250–257.

11 Chandna SM, Farrington K: Residual renal function: considerations on its importance and preservation in dialysis patients. Semin Dial 2004;17:196–201.

12 Lui SL, Cheng SW, Ng F, Ng SY, Wan KM, Yip T, Tse KC, Lam MF, Lai KN, Lo WK: Cefazolin plus netilmicin versus cefazolin plus ceftazidime for treating CAPD peritonitis: effect on residual renal function. Kidney Int 2005;68:2375–2380.

13 Antosiewicz S, Baczyński D, Wańkowicz Z: Does the treatment of peritonitis affect residual renal function in CAPD? Pol Arch Med Wewn 2001;106:1029–1033.

14 Mars RL, Moles K, Pope K, Hargrove P: Use of bolus intraperitoneal aminoglycosides for treating peritonitis in end-stage renal disease patients receiving continuous ambulatory peritoneal dialysis and continuous cycling peritoneal dialysis. Adv Perit Dial 2000;16: 280–284.

15 Murry KR, McKinnon PS, Mitrzyk B, Rybak MJ: Pharmacodynamic characterization of nephrotoxicity associated with once-daily aminoglycoside. Pharmacotherapy 1999;19: 1252–1260.

16 Rybak MJ, Abate BJ, Kang SL, Ruffing MJ, Lerner SA, Drusano GL: Prospective evaluation of the effect of an aminoglycoside dosing regimen on rates of observed nephrotoxicity and ototoxicity. Antimicrob Agents Chemother 1999;43:1549–1555.

17 Keller E: Peritoneal kinetics of different drugs. Clin Nephrol 1988;30(suppl 1): S24–S28.

18 Elwell RJ, Frye RF, Bailie GR: Pharmacokinetics of intraperitoneal cefepime in automated peritoneal dialysis. Perit Dial Int 2005;25:380–386.

19 Keller E: Peritoneal kinetics of different drugs. Clin Nephrol 1988;30:24–28.

20 Guay DR, Awni WM, Halstenson CE, Kenny MT, Keane WF, Matzke GR: Teicoplanin pharmacokinetics in patients undergoing continuous ambulatory peritoneal dialysis after intravenous and intraperitoneal dosing. Antimicrob Agents Chemother 1989;33: 2012–2015.

21 Stamatiadis D, Papaioannou MG, Giamarellos-Bourboulis EJ, Marinaki S, Giamarellou H, Stathakis CP: Pharmacokinetics of teicoplanin in patients undergoing continuous ambulatory peritoneal dialysis. Perit Dial Int 2003;23:127–131.

22 McIntosh ME, Smith WG, Junor BJ, Forrest G, Brodie MJ: Increased peritoneal permeability in patients with peritonitis undergoing continuous ambulatory peritoneal dialysis. Eur J Clin Pharmacol 1985;28:187–191.

23 Al-Wali W, Baillod RA, Brumfitt W, Hamilton-Miller JM: Intraperitoneal teicoplanin in CAPD peritonitis. Perit Dial Int 1990;10:107–108.

Sumio Hirata, PhD
Division of Clinical Pharmacology, Center for Clinical Pharmaceutical Sciences
Faculty of Pharmaceutical Sciences, Kumamoto University
5-1, Oe-Honmachi, Kumamoto 862-0973 (Japan)
Tel. +81 96 371 4856, E-Mail hirata@kumamoto-u.ac.jp

Suzuki H (ed): Home Dialysis in Japan.
Contrib Nephrol. Basel, Karger, 2012, vol 177, pp 38–47

Surgical and Medical Treatments of Encapsulation Peritoneal Sclerosis

Hideki Kawanishi

Tsuchiya General Hospital, Hiroshima, Japan

Abstract

Encapsulating peritoneal sclerosis (EPS) is a serious complication of long-term peritoneal dialysis (PD). The mortality rate for EPS has been high, primarily because of complications related to bowel obstruction. However, recent advances in clinical research have established the pathogenesis and course and a treatment strategy. To date, there is no consensus on therapy but care should be taken in trials using corticosteroid medication, and tamoxifen still remains controversial with respect to EPS treatment. The final therapeutic option for EPS is surgical enterolysis (adhesiolysis), and we have performed 239 surgical procedures in 181 patients and observed favorable outcomes. In the 1990s, Japan experienced a large number of EPS cases, and PD therapy faced a crisis. There were many negative viewpoints on treatment of EPS at the beginning, but surgery became accepted in the face of an increasing number of cases, and several other facilities introduced surgical therapy. This activity promoted the understanding of, and countermeasures against, EPS in Japan, and EPS is no longer recognized as a fatal complication.

In encapsulating peritoneal sclerosis (EPS), intraperitoneal inflammation leads to adhesive and inflammatory encapsulation of the intestinal tract, which then manifests as bowel obstruction syndrome. With the widespread use of peritoneal dialysis (PD), the number of patients developing EPS, a potentially fatal PD-related complication, has increased [1, 2]. As a consequence, there is much debate about whether there should be an arbitrary expiry date for PD because of the risk of EPS. However, recent clinical studies have clarified the pathogenesis of EPS and have proposed therapeutic strategies (table 1) [3].

In particular, the surgical option was previously contraindicated in patients with EPS [1]; however, the final option for patients in whom bowel obstruction symptoms fail to improve is surgical enterolysis, and we have actively performed

Table 1. Summary of alternatives for treatment and prevention of EPS [modified from ref. 3]

Prevention	
Minimize glucose concentration of prescribed PD solutions	Needs to be balanced against the need to avoid fluid overload
Minimize peritonitis incidence	Note that, frequently, EPS occurs in patients without a history of peritonitis
Perform post-PD peritoneal lavage	Retrospective study of peritoneal lavage confirmed the recovery of mesothelial cell surface area and prevention of EPS. Recommendation to higher risk case, i.e. long duration PD, high transporter, effluent markers
Use new PD solutions (neutral or physiologic pH, bicarbonate or bicarbonate, lactate buffer, non-glucose osmotic agents)	At present evidence is based either on in vitro indirect in vivo data. A multicenter study on the efficacy of this biocompatible PD fluid for the prevention of EPS is now under way
Identify predictive markers early	Identification of markers (i.e. PET, effluent-IL-6, -FDP, -CA125) may either guide modality selection at the pre-dialysis stage or allow for appropriate timing of withdrawal from PD
Treatment	
Total parenteral nutrition	Poor outcome as sole therapy; recommended as support for steroids and surgery
Corticosteroids	Recommend at pre-EPS, and inflammation stage. Timing is just onset of EPS
Tamoxifen	Prevention of peritoneal deterioration, observation study showed the decrease of mortality, still controversial to prevention and treatment for EPS
Surgery	Recent data indicate that surgical technique is of major importance for outcome (see present article)

this procedure since 1993. In EPS, the intestine is degenerated and vulnerable, and so the risk of intestinal perforation is high because of persistent obstruction. Such occurrences are fatal. We therefore consider that surgery is indicated for all EPS patients with severe symptoms of bowel obstruction [4–8].

Currently, understanding EPS is as follows: (1) EPS occurs after longer duration of PD, indicating the involvement of peritoneal deterioration; (2) EPS involves some kind of infection; (3) EPS frequently occurs after PD withdrawal and catheter removal; (4) timely administration of corticosteroids is effective, and (5) surgical enterolysis (adhesiolysis) is the optimal treatment to relieve bowel obstructions.

Pathogenesis of EPS

EPS develops when PD therapy (mainly with bioincompatible dialysis solutions) causes peritoneal deterioration, and a capsule formed by accumulated fibrin covers the deteriorated intestine and becomes firm, thereby impairing intestinal peristalsis, leading to the appearance of bowel obstruction symptoms [9]. The desquamation and disappearance of peritoneal mesothelial cells because of long-term exposure to PD solutions result in the progression of peritoneal fibrosis.

In addition, peritoneal capillary angiogenesis and hyperplasia develop, increasing peritoneal permeability [10]. The new vascular vessels appear to exhibit abnormally increased endothelial permeability to high molecular weight substances such as fibrin [9]. In this manner, a fibrin membrane is formed on the surface of a thickened, fibrotic peritoneum.

Fibrin deposited during PD is washed away with the dialysis solution, resulting in mild capsule formation. However, after PD withdrawal, fibrin remains in the abdominal cavity and accelerates capsule formation. In addition, a complicating inflammation, particularly bacterial peritonitis, further increases peritoneal permeability, and causes the deposition of large amounts of fibrin, leading to rapid capsule formation and EPS development. However, mild functional deterioration of the peritoneum does not lead to the development of EPS, because even when inflammation occurs and large amounts of fibrin deposit, no capsule is formed on the peritoneal surface. In contrast, in cases of severe peritoneal deterioration, even a slight inflammation easily leads to the formation of capsules, with the resulting development of EPS. Thus, EPS develops depending on the balance between the severity of peritoneal deterioration and that of inflammation [11].

Prevention

Development of EPS is based on deterioration of the peritoneum, and its rate of development is proportional to the duration of PD. Our prospective study showed that discontinuation of PD within 8 years reduces the risk of EPS development [2]. However, it is dangerous to prescribe the duration (in years) of PD, and it is necessary to evaluate the degree of peritoneal deterioration.

The simplest method of evaluation is the peritoneal equilibration test (PET) [12, 13]. If the patient is classified as a high transporter, PD should be discontinued. In addition, prevention of peritoneal deterioration is important to prevent the development of EPS. For this purpose, it is important to use biocompatible dialysis solutions to reduce the glucose load. Recently, a new neutral pH dialysis solution in a two-compartment bag has become available [14]. This solution contains smaller amounts of cytotoxic glucose degradation products and promises to prevent peritoneal deterioration.

Peritoneal Lavage: To remove fibrin, peritoneal lavage has been performed with a catheter left in place after withdrawal of PD. Retrospective study of peritoneal lavage confirmed the recovery of mesothelial cell surface area and prevention of EPS [15]. However, peritoneal lavage might not be expected to improve the deterioration of the peritoneum, only to prolong the time to thickening of the capsules, leading to the development of EPS. Peritonitis as a complication during peritoneal lavage has a reverse effect, inevitably leading to EPS.

In addition, it is problematic to physically stress a patient by leaving the catheter in place even after PD withdrawal, making it necessary to establish criteria to determine when to remove the catheter. In particular, there has been a recent trend towards performing peritoneal lavage in patients with a low risk of EPS, requiring strict indications for the procedure.

The indications for peritoneal lavage include: (1) long-term PD duration (>8 years); (2) peritoneal permeability increase diagnosed by PET; (3) increased levels of markers of inflammation, coagulation, fibrinolysis (IL-6, FDPs) in effluent, increased fibrin and/or protein in the effluent, a bloody effluent, and increase of mesothelial cells surface area. A PET is performed every 3 months during peritoneal lavage, and dialysate-to-plasma ratios of (D/P) creatinine, dialysate levels of cancer antigen-125 and mesothelial cells surface area are determined. If those values improve, the catheter should be removed [15, 16].

Treatment

Corticosteroids

Although steroids are currently the first-line drugs for the treatment of EPS, a prospective study showed that only 15 (38.5%) of 39 patients given steroids after EPS development achieved symptomatic improvement [2]. Steroids have the effect of suppressing inflammation to prevent ascites and fibrin deposition, but to be effective, they must be used immediately after EPS development [17, 18]. They are also effective in the pre-EPS stage when ascitic fluid increases. The timely administration of steroids terminates the inflammation and reduces ascitic fluid, thereby preventing progression to a state of bowel obstruction. However, delayed administration of steroids results in failure to prevent capsule formation, leading to the appearance of bowel obstruction symptoms. In rare cases, the administration of steroids is effective, but dose reduction results in recurrence in some patients. Their treatment poses a challenge, requiring careful dose reduction. If an effect is achieved, the dose should be continued for a long period.

Steroids cannot be expected to be effective for EPS associated with established bowel obstruction symptoms. If the CRP level is persistently elevated, steroid administration is continued, but gradually tapered, and surgical treatment is considered, as will be described shortly.

Is prophylactic steroid administration effective? The indications include: (1) inflammatory cell infiltration confirmed by peritoneal biopsy before EPS development; (2) persistent CRP positivity in the absence of other infections; (3) a rapid increase in ascitic fluid, and (4) an increase in markers of inflammation, coagulation, and fibrinolysis (such as IL-6 and FDPs) in the effluent. However, it has not been demonstrated that prophylactic steroid administration prevents the development of EPS. In any event, steroids should been administered following strict indications.

Tamoxifen

Tamoxifen is a non-steroidal anti-estrogen used to treat carcinoma of the breast. It is also used in treating fibrosing diseases such as fibrosing medianitis and retroperitoneal fibrosis. The administration of tamoxifen has been attempted mainly in Europe for the prevention of peritoneal fibrosis. However, its effectiveness remains unclear because of the limited number of patients [19–21]. The proposed mechanism of action of tamoxifen is that it upregulates transforming growth factor-β_1, which stimulates metalloproteinase-9 to remove degenerated collagen, thereby preventing damage to mesothelial cells [19]. A recent study of immunophenotyping of peritoneal biopsy specimens includes EPS cases that showed the sparse expression of estrogen receptor of the peritoneal [22]. Thus, the blockade of the estrogen receptor of tamoxifen is probably not the mechanism of action.

In the Dutch Multicentre EPS Study, EPS was retrospectively analyzed in 63 patients and the efficacy of survival rate of tamoxifen was presented; the mortality rate in the tamoxifen group (n = 24) was 45.8% compared to the non-tamoxifen group (n = 39) that was 63.5% (p < 0.077) [23]. However, the large retrospective Pan-Thames EPS Study could not define the effectiveness of medical treatment with tamoxifen [24]. Tamoxifen is administered at daily doses of 10–20 mg and care should be taken in increasing the dose because of the frequent development of complicating thrombotic lesions [21]. From these findings, tamoxifen is still controversial with respect to the prevention and treatment of EPS. Larger prospective studies are necessary to confirm the effects of such medication.

Surgical Options

Our first encounter with an EPS patient who underwent surgical enterolysis (adhesiolysis) was in 1993; that patient was completely cured. From then until the end of 2010, we performed 239 enterolysis procedures in 181 patients [8]. Of these 181 patients, 14 died after surgery; the others all showed improvement.

Considering the mechanism of EPS development, the surgical technique is simple, involving only the division of peritoneal adhesions by repeated lysis of fibrin membranes with a sharp instrument (fig. 1). Recently, to identify the site of stenosis, we have, after enterolysis, been inserting a Miller-Abbott ileus tube with an inflated balloon to the end of the ileum.

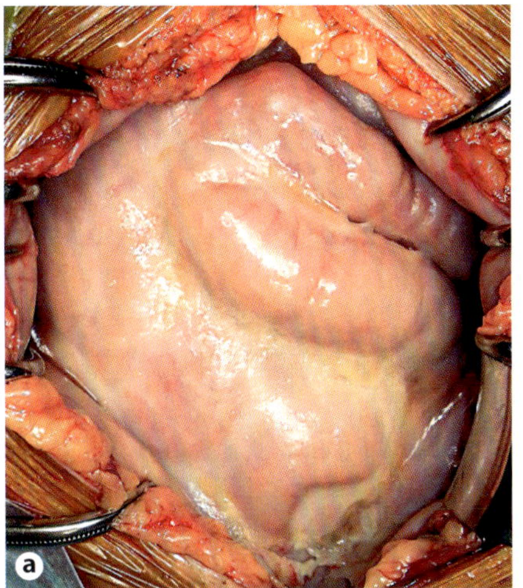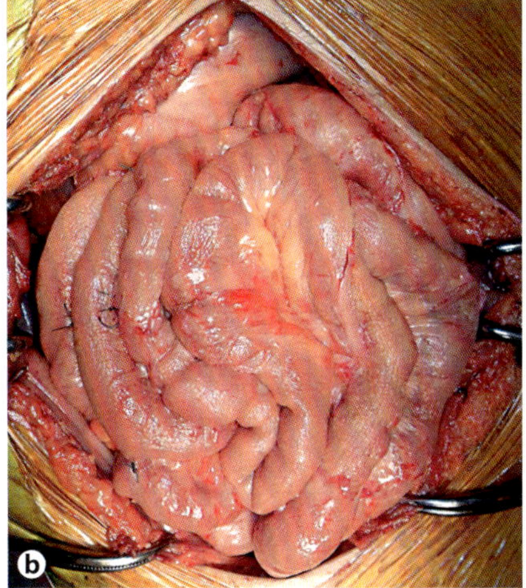

Fig. 1. Finding at laparotomy (**a**) in a patient with EPS and after complete enterolysis (**b**).

Surgery can reverse the bowel obstruction, but it does not improve the peritoneal deterioration. As a result, the capsules can re-form, and EPS can recur in some patients 6–12 months later. In addition, adhesions also occur as a result of surgical injury to the intestinal wall and mesenteric serosa. To prevent recurrences, we have, since April 2007, been performing the Noble plication procedure [25, 26], in which intestine is sutured to intestine to prevent re-obstruction of the bowel. This technique prevents not only passage disturbances resulting from kinking and adhesion of the small intestine, but also escape into and adhesions in the pelvic cavity. Patients experiencing recurrence or presenting difficulties in complete adhesiolysis because of intestinal wall calcification require a bypass between the oral site jejunum and the ileum or large intestine.

Surgical Results
Most of the 14 patients (7.7%) who died postoperatively died of sepsis resulting from intestinal perforation and infection; 1 died from hepatic failure. Enterolysis was performed in 169 first surgeries; the Noble plication was added in 57 recent cases. Bypass between the oral site jejunum and the ileum or large intestine was performed in 9 patients in whom enterolysis could not be performed. In 3 patients with localized adhesions and mild degeneration of the wall of the small intestine, the adhered small intestine was resected and anastomosed.

Of 112 patients treated solely with enterolysis in the first surgery, 34 (30.4%) required re-surgery. In 57 patients, enterolysis with Noble plication was performed in the first surgery; 7 of these patients (12.3%) required re-surgery. We compared the course of re-surgery between patients who underwent the Noble plication procedure and those who underwent enterolysis alone for their initial

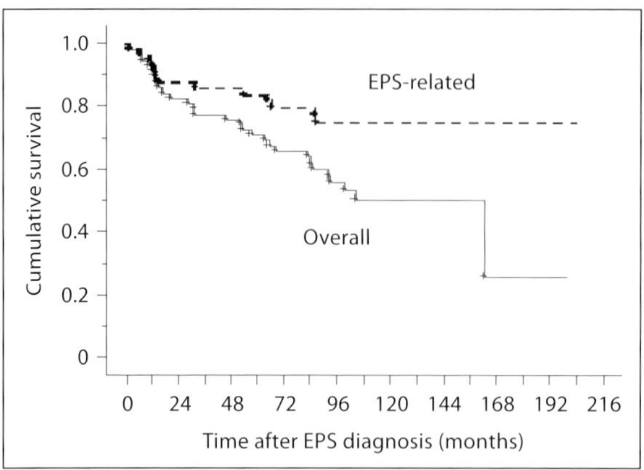

Fig. 2. Kaplan-Maier survival curve in EPS after surgical options, contrasting overall outcomes and EPS-related outcomes for 1993–2010.

surgery. Although a long-term comparison is difficult because the follow-up period for the Noble plication group is short, the 1- and 2-year rates of freedom from a re-surgery are higher in the group treated with Noble plication (0.91 vs. 0.76 and 0.81 vs. 0.70 respectively), suggesting that the Noble plication is effective in preventing recurrence [8].

Outcomes of Surgical Options
At the end of 2010, outcomes in 6 of the 181 patients were unknown. Excluding those 6 patients, the mean duration of postoperative follow-up was 46.4 months (range 0.3–208 months). A total of 64 patients who opted for surgery (35.4%) died. Death was related to EPS in 33 patients (18.2%), including the 14 who died postoperatively (table 1). The overall survival rate at 1, 2, 3, 5, and 8 years after diagnosis was 93, 83, 78, 71, and 60% respectively. The survival rate for non-EPS-related death at 1, 2, 3, 5, and 8 years after diagnosis was 95, 90, 87, 81, and 74% respectively (fig. 2) [8].

Recommendation of Surgical Options
Previously, the literature contained only case reports of the use of the surgical option for EPS [27–29]. Surgery was previously contraindicated in patients with EPS, and most patients treated surgically died of peritonitis as a postoperative complication [1]. These deaths occurred because the pathogenesis of EPS was not well understood by surgeons, and in many cases, simple resection of adherent intestinal loops with enteroanastomosis was performed by surgeons who had never been involved with PD.

We developed a surgical technique of total intestinal enterolysis without enterectomy and since have treated patients in the belief that surgical therapy is the only curative treatment for established EPS [4–8]. In the period between

Table 2. Comparison of outcomes in EPS from recent studies

Study	Patients n	Follow-up years	Overall mortality, %	Survival rate, %			
				1st year	2nd year	3rd year	5th year
Pan-Thames EPS Study [24]	111	11	53	56	50		
ANZDATA Registry [30]	33	13	55	69	62	58	35
Dutch Multicentre EPS Study [23]	64	12.7					
Tamoxifen			45.8	80	75	60	
No tamoxifen			74.4	63	52	40	
Surgical option Kawanishi et al. [8]	181	17	35.4	93	83	78	71

1993 and the end of 2010, we performed 239 enterolysis procedures in 181 patients. Of these 181 patients, 14 died after surgery; the others all showed improvement.

The mortality rate from EPS has been reported to be 24–66%, but findings lack clarity because of variations in the follow-up periods and treatment methods. The results of a relatively long-term follow-up have recently been reported. In the Pan-Thames EPS Study, in which EPS was observed in 111 patients, the overall mortality and 1-year overall survival rates were 53 and 56% respectively [24]. In the Australia and New Zealand Dialysis and Transplant Registry, the overall mortality rate in 33 EPS patients was 55%, and the 1-, 2-, 3-, and 5-year survival rates were 69, 62, 58, and 35% respectively [30]. In the Dutch Multicentre EPS Study, EPS was retrospectively analyzed in 63 patients, and the efficacy of tamoxifen was presented, but the overall mortality rate was 63.5%, and the 1-, 2-, and 3-year survival rates in the tamoxifen group (24 patients with an overall mortality rate of 45.8%) were 80, 75, and 60% respectively [23]. Compared with these recent reports the outcomes in our study were markedly favorable: the overall mortality rate was 35.4% and the 1-, 2-, 3-, and 5-year survival rates were 93, 83, 78, and 71% respectively (table 2).

Given that the observation period in our study was 17 years, the severity of EPS may have changed, and the surgical techniques have been modified. Moreover, the therapeutic results were collected at a single facility and therefore cannot be directly compared with results collected at multiple facilities. However, the usefulness of surgical therapy for EPS has not been ruled out because all surgeries were performed by the same operator and surgical team under a set therapeutic policy.

Conclusions

In the 1990s, Japan experienced a large number of EPS cases, and PD therapy faced a crisis [1]. There were many negative viewpoints on the surgical treatment of EPS at the beginning, but surgery became accepted in the face of an increasing number of cases, and several other facilities introduced surgical therapy. This activity promoted the understanding of, and countermeasures against, EPS in Japan, and EPS is no longer recognized as a fatal complication. To improve the surgical results, a surgical team with a thorough understanding of the pathology of EPS is essential, for which the establishment of a regional EPS treatment center in each community and the training of surgeons are necessary.

In addition, biocompatible PD fluid (fluid low in glucose degradation products) became available for all patients, which may have reduced the EPS risk. A multicenter study on the efficacy of this biocompatible PD fluid for the prevention of EPS is now under way [31].

References

1 Nomoto Y, Kawaguchi Y, Kubo H, et al: Sclerosing encapsulating peritonitis in patients undergoing continuous ambulatory peritoneal dialysis: a report of the Japanese Sclerosing Encapsulating Peritonitis Study Group. Am J Kidney Dis 1996;28:420–427.

2 Kawanishi H, Kawaguchi Y, Fukui H, et al: Encapsulating peritoneal sclerosis in Japan: a prospective, controlled, multicenter study. Am J Kidney Dis 2004;44:729–737.

3 Kawaguchi Y, Saito A, Kawanishi H, et al: Recommendations on the management of encapsulating peritoneal sclerosis in Japan, 2005: diagnosis, predictive markers, treatment, and preventive measures. Perit Dial Int 2005;25(suppl 4):S83–S95.

4 Kawanishi H, Harada Y, Sakikubo E, et al: Surgical treatment for sclerosing encapsulating peritonitis. Adv Perit Dial 2000;16: 252–256.

5 Kawanishi H, Watanabe H, Moriishi M, et al: Successful surgical management of encapsulating peritoneal sclerosis. Perit Dial Int 2005;25(suppl 4):S39–S47.

6 Kawanishi H, Moriishi M, Tsuchiya S: Experience of 100 surgical cases of encapsulating peritoneal sclerosis: investigation of recurrent cases after surgery. Adv Perit Dial 2006;22:60–64.

7 Kawanishi H, Ide K, Yamashita M, et al: Surgical techniques for prevention of recurrence after total enterolysis in encapsulating peritoneal sclerosis. Adv Perit Dial 2008;24: 51–55.

8 Kawanishi H, Shintaku S, Moriishi M, et al: Seventeen years' experience of surgical options for encapsulating peritoneal sclerosis. Adv Perit Dial 2011;27:53–58.

9 Dobbie JW: Pathogenesis of peritoneal fibrosing syndromes (sclerosing peritonitis) in peritoneal dialysis. Perit Dial Int 1992;12: 14–27.

10 De Vriese AS, Tilton RG, Stephan CC, et al: Vascular endothelial growth factor is essential for hyperglycemia-induced structural and functional alterations of the peritoneal membrane. J Am Soc Nephrol 2001;12: 1734–1741.

11 Kawanishi H, Harada Y, Noriyuki T, et al: Treatment options for encapsulating peritoneal sclerosis based on progressive stage. Adv Perit Dial 2001;17:200–204.

12 Yamamoto R, Nakayama M, Hasegawa T, et al: High-transport membrane is a risk factor for encapsulating peritoneal sclerosis developing after long-term continuous ambulatory peritoneal dialysis treatment. Adv Perit Dial 2002;18:131–134.

13 Lambie ML, John B, Mushahar L, et al: The peritoneal osmotic conductance is low well before the diagnosis of encapsulating peritoneal sclerosis is made. Kidney Int 2010;78:611–618.

14 Williams JD, Topley N, Craig KJ, et al: The Euro-Balance Trial: the effect of a new biocompatible peritoneal dialysis fluid (balance) on the peritoneal membrane. Kidney Int 2004;66:408–418.

15 Yamamoto T, Nagasue K, Okuno S, et al: The role of peritoneal lavage and the prognostic significance of mesothelial cell area in preventing encapsulating peritoneal sclerosis. Perit Dial Int 2010;30:343–352

16 Moriishi M, Kawanishi H, Kawai T, et al: Preservation of peritoneal catheter for prevention of encapsulating peritoneal sclerosis. Adv Perit Dial 2002;18:149–153.

17 Junor BJ, McMillan MA: Immunosuppression in sclerosing peritonitis. Adv Perit Dial 1993;9:187–189.

18 Mori Y, Tatsuo S, Sutoh H, et al: A case of a dialysis patient with sclerosing peritonitis successfully treated with corticosteroid therapy alone. Am J Kidney Dis 1997;30:275–278.

19 Allaria PM, Giangrande A, Gandini E, et al: Continuous ambulatory peritoneal dialysis and sclerosing encapsulating peritonitis: tamoxifen as a new therapeutic agent? J Nephrol 1999;12:395–397.

20 Eltoum MA, Wright S, Atchley J, et al: Four consecutive cases of peritoneal dialysis–related encapsulating peritoneal sclerosis treated successfully with tamoxifen. Perit Dial Int 2006;26:203–206.

21 Del Peso G, Bajo MA, Gil F, et al: Clinical experience with tamoxifen in peritoneal fibrosing syndromes. Adv Perit Dial 2003;19:32–35.

22 Braun N, Fritz P, Biegger D, et al: Difference in the expression of hormone receptors and fibrotic markers in the human peritoneum – implications for therapeutic targets to prevent encapsulating peritoneal sclerosis. Perit Dial Int 2011;31:291–300.

23 Korte MR, Fieren MW, Sampimon DE, et al, on behalf of the investigators of the Dutch Multicentre EPS Study: Tamoxifen is associated with lower mortality of encapsulating peritoneal sclerosis: results of the Dutch Multicentre EPS Study. Nephrol Dial Transplant 2011;26:691–697.

24 Balasubramaniam G, Brown EA, Davenport A, et al: The Pan-Thames EPS Study: treatment and outcomes of encapsulating peritoneal sclerosis. Nephrol Dial Transplant 2009;24:3209–3215.

25 Noble TB Jr: Plication of small intestine as prophylaxis against adhesions. Am J Surg 1937;35:41–44.

26 Seabrook DB, Wilson ND: Prevention and treatment of intestinal obstruction by use of the Noble procedure. Am J Surg 1954;88:186–193.

27 Jackson BT: Surgical treatment of sclerosing peritonitis caused by practolol. Br J Surg 1977;64:255–257.

28 Smith L, Collins JF, Morris M, et al: Sclerosing encapsulating peritonitis associated with continuous ambulatory peritoneal dialysis: surgical management. Am J Kidney Dis 1997;29:456–460.

29 Assalia A, Schein M, Hashmonai M: Problems in the surgical management of sclerosing encapsulating peritonitis. Isr J Med Sci 1993;29:686–688.

30 Johnson DW, Cho Y, Livingston BE, et al: Encapsulating peritoneal sclerosis: incidence, predictors, and outcomes. Kidney Int 2010;77:904–912.

31 Kawanishi H, Nakayama M, Miyazaki M, et al, for the NEXT-PD Study Group: Prospective multicenter observational study of encapsulating peritoneal sclerosis with neutral dialysis solution – the NEXT-PD study. Adv Perit Dial 2010;26:71–74.

Hideki Kawanishi, MD
Tsuchiya General Hospital
3-30 Nakajima-cho, Naka-ku
Hiroshima 730-8655 (Japan)
Tel. +81 82 243 9191, E-Mail h-kawanishi@tsuchiya-hp.jp

Suzuki H (ed): Home Dialysis in Japan.
Contrib Nephrol. Basel, Karger, 2012, vol 177, pp 48–56

Application of Peritoneal Dialysis in Elderly Patients by Classifying the Age into Young-Old, Old, and Oldest-Old

Makoto Hiramatsu[a] · Mari Ishida[b] · Yukio Tonozuka[c] · Hiroko Mikami[a] · Toshio Yamanari[a] · Noriya Momoki[a] · Akifumi Onishi[a] · Keisuke Maruyama[a]

[a]Okayama Saiseikai General Hospital, Okayama, [b]Jinyukai Kitasaito Hospital, Asahikawa, and [c]Baxter Ltd, Tokyo, Japan

Abstract

Background: A greater number of end-stage renal disease patients are receiving peritoneal dialysis (PD) or hemodialysis (HD) in Japan. However, medical concerns with advancing age have been raised in PD utilization for elderly patients. The objective of this study was to address the indications for PD in elderly patients in terms of medical concerns such as nutrition state, residual renal function, dialysis efficiency, peritonitis, cardiovascular disease (CVD) complications, and technique survival. **Methods:** In a retrospective, two-center study, we evaluated 247 patients who newly started PD from 2002 to 2008. All patients were divided into four groups: young (<64 years, n = 99), young-old (65–74 years, n = 55), old (75–84 years, n = 62) and oldest-old (≥85 years, n = 31). Serum albumin, hemoglobin, β_2-microglobulin, cardio-thoracic ratio, 24-hour urine collection and spent dialysate volume was collected at the initiation of PD and after 1, 2, 3, and 4 years. PD withdrawal, occurrence of CVD complications, peritonitis and death were recorded. **Results:** Nephrosclerosis as a primary disease increased with advancing age (p = 0.001). At baseline, gender, body weight, serum creatinine, hemoglobin and cardio-thoracic ratio were significantly different among the four groups. No significant decrease was shown in urine output with advancing age. The spent dialysate volume was significantly lower (mean 3.8 liters/day) in the oldest-old group compared with the other groups (p = 0.001). However, a smaller volume of PD fluid in the oldest-old group was not accompanied by a significantly higher serum β_2-microgloblin level compared with the other groups and there was no reason of PD withdrawal for underdialysis in the old and oldest-old groups. Neither the incidence of CVD complications nor that of peritonitis was increased with advancing age. There was no significant difference in technique survival rate excluding death between each group. These findings suggest that there are no medical concerns to avoid PD therapy in elderly end-stage renal disease patients.

The age of patients requiring dialysis for the renal replacement therapy is increasing year by year and the number of elderly patients receiving dialysis is also growing steadily. Patients over 65 years account for about 60% or more of the patients who are started on dialysis in Japan. The prevalence of peritoneal dialysis (PD) is 3.4% and it is reported that 4.2% of end-stage renal disease patients in the over 90-year group initiated PD therapy [1]. Moreover, PD has a certain number of benefits compared to hemodialysis (HD). Some of these advantages are the absence of vascular access, longer preservation of residual renal function and better hemodynamic tolerance. Others have more social characteristics, such as home treatment and the possibility of outpatient nursing care assistance. Therefore, PD therapy could be suitable for the elderly patients in view of their physical, mental, and social characteristics. However, medical concerns about PD therapy for elderly patients have never been fully studied in a population stratified by age: 'young old' of 65–74 years, 'old' of 75–84, and 'oldest-old' of ≥85. Initiation of PD for the very old poses several age-related medical concerns, including malnutrition, onset of peritonitis, increased prevalence of cardiovascular diseases (CVD), and decreased rate of treatment compliance. The objective of this study was to retrospectively investigate the nutritional status, urine output, dialysis efficiency, CVD complications, occurrence of peritonitis and the rate of technical survival in elderly patients subjected to PD, and to assess the medical concerns in different age groups.

Methods

This is a retrospective study in two hospitals. We evaluated 247 patients who newly started PD between January 2002 and December 2008 at Okayama Saiseikai General Hospital (n = 109) and Kitasaito Hospital (n = 138). Inclusion criteria were age >18 years and survival >1 month. We extracted patient's sex, age upon starting of PD, type of PD, and primary disease. All patients were divided into four groups: young (<64 years, n = 99), young-old (65–74 years, n = 55), old (75–84 years, n = 62) and oldest-old (≥85 years, n = 31). Serum albumin, hemoglobin, β_2-microglobulin, CRP, triglyceride, creatinine, cardio-thoracic ratio (CTR), 24-hour urine collection and spent dialysate volume was collected at the initiation of PD and after 1, 2, 3, and 4 years. All laboratory samples were analyzed in the each hospital by standard laboratory techniques. PD withdrawal, occurrence of CVD complications, peritonitis and death were recorded. Peritonitis episodes were expressed classically as the peritonitis rate of one episode per patient-month and CVD disease was defined as the presence of ischemic heart disease, myocardial infraction, a cerebrovascular event or peripheral vascular disease for each age group. Patients were censored at transfer to another dialysis unit and lost to follow-up. Continuous variables were described by means and standard deviations; categorical variables were described as frequencies and percentages. Statistical significance was accepted for $p \leq 0.05$. Differences between groups were assessed by χ^2 test and ANOVA. All statistical analyses were performed with SPSS software (version 17.0; SPSS, Inc., Chicago, Ill., USA).

Results

Clinical Background in Four Groups
We examined 247 PD patients who were divided into the four groups: young, young-old, old, and oldest-old (table 1). As for primary diseases, diabetic nephropathy accounted for 48 and 41% in the young and young-old groups, respectively, showing a significant difference with the other groups (p = 0.001). On the other hand, nephrosclerosis accounted for 55 and 69% in the old and oldest-old groups, respectively, also showing a significant difference compared with the other groups (p = 0.001). This result indicated that the proportion of diabetic nephropathy decreased and the ratio of nephrosclerosis increased with advancing age. The ratio of gender was higher in men of the young group, equal in men and women of the old group, and significantly higher in women of the oldest-old group, showing an increasing tendency with advancing age in women. As for the modality selection of continuous ambulatory peritoneal dialysis (CAPD) and automated peritoneal dialysis (APD), there was no difference among the age groups. Though APD therapy needs mechanical procedures for the patients or caregivers, APD was selected in 44 and 37% of the patients in the old and oldest-old groups respectively. Body weight significantly decreased (p = 0.001) and CTR significantly increased with advancing age (p = 0.001). Serum creatinine and hemoglobin levels significantly decreased with aging, while total cholesterol and triglycerides showed no significant changes in the four groups.

Residual Renal Function
It is reported that residual renal function and urine output are advantageously maintained by PD compared with HD [2–6], resulting in improvement of the survival and quality of life of the patients, and avoidance of complications [2]. The daily urine output, which was used as an index of residual renal function, was at the initiation of PD 796.8 ± 458.5, 828.3 ± 453.7, 888.9 ± 528.5, and 772.5 ± 435.3 ml/day on average in the young, young old, old, and oldest-old groups, respectively. There was no significant difference among the groups. After 4 years on PD the urine output was 533.3 ± 486.9, 468.9 ± 332.7, 711.4 ± 593.5, and 550.0 ± 353.6 ml/day on average in the young, young-old, old and oldest-old groups, respectively. In all the age groups, including the oldest-old, nearly 500 ml/day of urine output was maintained for 4 years (fig. 1). The 4-year comparison of urine output among the age groups showed no significant differences.

Change of Serum Albumin
Albumin was considered as a surrogate for nutritional state [7, 8]. Moreover, serum albumin levels of PD patients have been reported to affect their survival [9]. In PD, proteins are lost from the peritoneal cavity and this is a

Table 1. Baseline characteristic in four groups

	Young	Young-old	Old	Oldest-old	p value
Patients, n	99	55	62	31	
Age	52.0±10.8	70.1±2.9	79.7±2.8	90.0±3.3	0.001[b]
Female/male	33/65	20/35	31/31	24/7	0.001[a]
Primary disease (diabetic nephropathy/non-diabetic nephropathy)	45/47	22/30	14/37	2/26	0.00[a]
Primary disease (nephrosclerosis/non-nephrosclerosis)	5/87	11/41	29/22	20/8	0.001[a]
CAPD/APD	53/35	29/18	31/24	19/11	0.919[a]
Body weight, kg	61.6±10.6	56.9±12.6	50.9±10.8	45.2±7.4	0.001[b]
CTR, %	48.1±5.1	51.2±5.0	51.9±5.9	57.9±6.4	0.001[b]
Serum albumin, g/dl	3.4±0.6	3.1±0.9	3.1±0.5	2.8±0.5	0.001[b]
Serum creatinine, mg/dl	8.0±3.0	6.5±2.5	6.5±2.4	5.8±2.5	0.001[b]
BUN, mg/dl	59.1±23.7	56.5±17.2	67.6±84.9	60.0±22.9	0.597[b]
Hemoglobin, g/dl	9.4±1.7	9.6±1.4	8.8±1.7	8.8±2.0	0.043[b]
Hematocrit, %	28.3±4.8	29.1±4.0	27.6±4.1	27.7±4.4	0.293[b]
Total cholesterol, mg/dl	173.9±51.8	175.4±54.3	162.2±39.0	162.2±42.6	0.312[b]
LDL cholesterol, mg/dl	102.8±44.7	103.5±48.4	91.1±33.0	99.3±31.6	0.42[b]
HDL cholesterol, mg/dl	45.5±22.2	41.9±18.9	41.9±17.1	36.2±11.4	0.185[b]
Triglycerides, mg/dl	139.6±100.3	138.6±81.5	114.9±47.8	113.7±84.4	0.195[b]
CRP, mg/dl	0.5±1.1	1.3±2.5	0.5±0.6	1.6±2.7	0.037[b]
White blood cells, /mm^3	5191.9±2602.1	4714.3±2981.0	4659.9±2718.2	5357.7±2729.0	0.474[b]
β_2-Microgloblin, mg/l	16.9±6.5	17.6±6.4	18.1±5.8	20.0±5.1	0.259[b]
Systolic blood pressure, mm Hg	140.8±21.9	132.5±25.0	132.0±22.8	132.0±25.3	0.064[b]
Diastolic blood pressure, mm Hg	80.7±13.5	72.8±14.7	70.6±15.0	66.7±13.1	0.001[b]
PD duration, days	838.2±565.3	751.2±694.0	611.5±547.2	597.4±509.1	0.058[b]
Urine output, ml/day	796.8±458.5	828.3±453.7	888.9±528.5	772.5±435.3	0.688[b]

[a] Between groups χ^2 test.
[b] Between groups ANOVA.

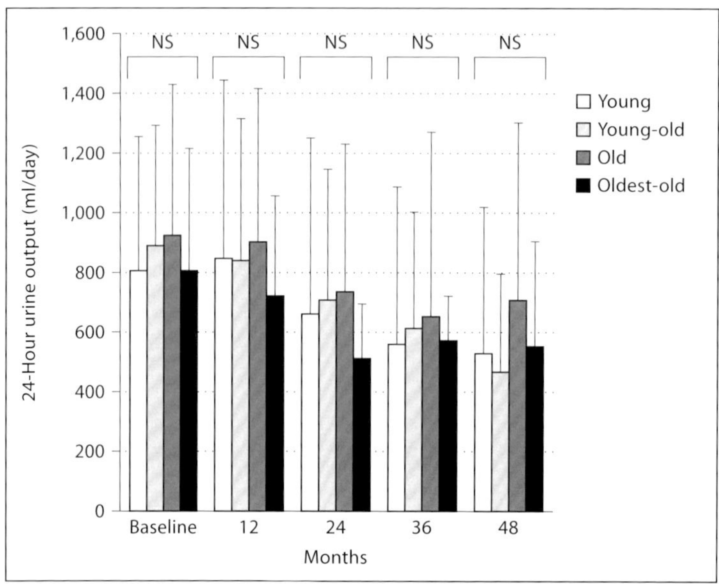

Fig. 1. 24-Hour urine output in elderly patients.

matter of concern, especially in elderly patients with poor appetite. Therefore, we compared serum albumin levels in the four age groups and analyzed the changes during 4 years. The results showed that serum albumin levels at the initiation of PD were 3.4 ± 0.6, 3.1 ± 0.6, and 3.1 ± 0.5 g/dl on average in the young, young-old, and old groups, respectively, with no significant differences among them. However, in the oldest-old group, serum albumin level was 2.8 ± 0.5 g/dl on average, which was significantly lower than that in the other groups. After 1, 2, 3, and 4 years of PD, we likewise examined serum albumin levels and found that the oldest-old group showed a significantly lower level of serum albumin compared with the other three groups at each time period (p = 0.001) (data not shown). Nevertheless, the investigation of successive changes in serum albumin levels in the oldest-old group did not show a significant decrease within the same group for 4 years in the study period. This result indicated that serum albumin levels did not change during treatment of PD in the oldest-old group.

Comparison of Clinical Outcome
As for the occurrence of cardiovascular events and peritonitis, and the rate of technical survival during the study, CVD events occurred in 19.2, 14.5, 8.0, and 22.6% of the patients in the young, young old, old, and oldest-old groups, respectively. There were no significant changes related to the onset of CVD in each age group. The onset of peritonitis was 69.7, 82.9, 63.3, and 324.9 per

	Young	Young-old	Old	Oldest-old	p value
CVD rate	19/80 (19.2%)	8/47 (14.5%)	5/57 (8.0%)	7/24 (22.6%)	0.188[a]
Peritonitis rate	22/77 (22.2%)	9/46 (16.3%)	14/48 (22.6%)	2/29 (6.5%)	0.204[a]
Peritonitis, patient-months	69.7	82.9	63.3	324.9	
Technique survival excluding death	49/43 (47.7%)	17/22 (56.4%)	17/17 (50.0%)	2/6 (75.0%)	0.395[a]
24-Hour spent dialysate volume, l/day	6.3±2.0	5.7±1.7	5.0±1.6	3.8±1.2[b]	0.001[c]

[a] Between groups χ^2 test.
[b] Differs from all other groups.
[c] Between groups ANOVA.

patient-month in the young, young-old, old, and oldest-old groups, respectively, and the incidence of peritonitis did not increase with advancing age. The rate of technical survival, excluding death, showed 47.7, 56.4, 50.0, and 75.0% in the young, young-old, old, and oldest-old groups, respectively, showing no significant differences among the groups. These results showed that advancing age did not relate with the proportion of withdrawal from PD treatment (table 2).

Peritoneal Dialysate Volume and Dialysis Efficiency
Table 2 shows usage of peritoneal dialysate volume per day at the initiation of PD. The spent dialysate volume gradually decreases with advancing age. The average of peritoneal dialysate volume was the highest in the young group (6.3 ± 2.0 liters/day). In the young old, old, and oldest-old groups it was 5.7 ± 1.7, 5.0 ± 1.6, and 3.8 ± 1.2 liters/day on average, respectively. The volume of peritoneal dialysate in the oldest-old group was significantly lower compared with that in the other three groups (oldest-old vs. young, p = 0.001; oldest-old vs. young-old, p = 0.001; oldest-old vs. old, p = 0.012). This result suggested that usage of peritoneal dialysate volume decreased with advancing age. However, smaller volumes of peritoneal dialysate may cause inadequacy of dialysis for the elderly patients. To address this issue, as an index of dialysis efficiency, changes of serum β_2-microglobulin levels were compared during 4 years in the four groups. β_2-Microglobulin levels gradually increased at a successive time point: PD initiation, 1, 2, 3, and 4 years. However, there were no significant differences among the four groups at each time point (fig. 2). These results suggested that a smaller volume of peritoneal dialysate in the oldest-old group was not accompanied by a significantly higher serum β_2-microgloblin level compared with other groups. Also, there was no significant difference in technique survival rate excluding death between each group.

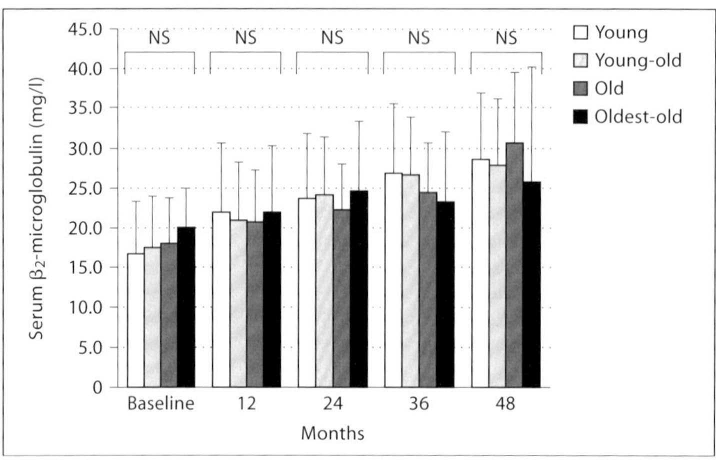

Fig. 2. Concentration of serum β_2-microglobulin in elderly patients.

Discussion

It is thought that avoiding physical burden and maintaining residual renal function are important to prevent complications and improve survival rates of elderly patients for dialysis therapy [10–13] and PD is more beneficial than HD to maintain residual renal function [2–6]. We previously reported that preservation of residual renal function was better in elderly patients aged ≥70 compared with those <70 years old [14]. In this study, sufficient urine output of around 500 ml/day was found in each group during 4 years suggesting that elderly patients benefit from PD therapy, that is maintenance of residual renal function. However, initiation of PD in elderly patients often raises various medical concerns related to advancing age, including increased occurrence of peritonitis and lower technical survival, due to difficulties during the PD procedure, and loss of albumin from the peritoneal cavity. Regarding these concerns, this study showed the following results: (1) urine output was well maintained, (2) occurrence of peritonitis and CVD events did not increase, (3) the rate of technical survival did not decrease, and (4) serum albumin levels did not decline over time. Therefore, it was suggested that the merit of PD could be maintained in the case of elderly patients. Furthermore, the benefits of PD for elderly people include the gradual decrease of PD dialysate volume per day with advancing age. The number of peritoneal dialysate volumes used in the oldest-old group was significantly smaller than that in the other age groups. In order to examine if the decrease in the number of PD bags might cause inadequate dialysis, 4-year changes in β_2-microglobulin, as an indicator of adequacy of dialysis, were analyzed. The results showed no significant

     Hiramatsu · Ishida · Tonozuka · Mikami · Yamanari · Momoki · Onishi · Maruyama increase of β_2-microglobulin with advancing age, which was considered to be caused by a decreased basal metabolism and the smaller physique of the elderly. Especially old and oldest-old patients could undergo PD with a smaller volume of dialysate and no withdrawal from PD due to inadequate dialysis occurring in both groups. Moreover, it is also considered that usage of a smaller volume of peritoneal dialysate is beneficial to avoid excessive albumin loss from the peritoneal cavity as far as possible. The lower frequency of bag exchange for the elderly compared with that in the younger patients is beneficial not only for the patients themselves but also for the home dialysis caregivers, and suggests that PD is suitable for elderly patients, especially old and oldest-old patients.

The results of this study indicate that there are not too many medical concerns regarding initiation of PD in the elderly. Also, previous comparative studies on PD and HD in elderly patients suggested that PD was more appropriate for them for the following reasons: impact of dialysis on the cardiovascular system was low, more freedom of diet was obtained because of relatively long maintenance of residual renal function with less fluid restriction, the advantages of PD as home dialysis decreased transfer to a hospital than HD, and reduced physical burden and quality of life could be improved [15–18]. Even based on the results of this study, however, independence of patients and family support are indispensable for initiation of PD therapy in the elderly. Advancing age itself is not necessarily disadvantageous for the implementation of PD.

Conclusion

The findings in our study, in which elderly patients were classified as young, young-old, old and oldest-old, suggest that there are no medical concerns to avoid PD therapy in elderly end-stage renal disease patients.

Acknowledgment

We are grateful to all patients and medical staffs participating in this study.

References

1 Nakai S, Suzuki K, Masakane I, Wada A, Itami N, Ogata S, Kimata N, Shigematsu T, Shinoda T, Syouji T, Taniguchi M, Tsuchida K, Nakamoto H, Nishi S, Nishi H, Hashimoto S, Hasegawa T, Hanafusa N, Hamano T, Fujii N, Marubayashi S, Morita O, Yamagata K, Wakai K, Watanabe Y, Iseki K, Tsubakihara Y: Renal Data Registry Committee, Japanese Society for Dialysis Therapy, Tokyo, Japan. Overview of regular dialysis treatment in Japan. Ther Apher Dial 2010;14:505–540.

2 Perl J, Bargman JM: The importance of residual kidney function for patients on dialysis: a critical review. Am J Kidney Dis 2009;53:1068–1081.

3 Jansen MA, Hart AA, Korevaar JC, Dekker FW, Boeschoten EW, Krediet RT, NECOSAD Study Group: Predictors of the rate of decline of residual renal function in incident dialysis patients. Kidney Int 2002;62:1046–1053.

4 Moist LM, Port FK, Orzol SM, Young EW, Ostbye T, Wolfe RA, Hulbert-Shearon T, Jones CA, Bloembergen WE: Predictors of loss of residual renal function among new dialysis patients. J Am Soc Nephrol 2000;11:556–564.

5 Misra M, Vonesh E, Van Stone JC, Moore HL, Prowant B, Nolph KD: Effect of cause and time of dropout on the residual GFR: a comparative analysis of the decline of GFR on dialysis. Kidney Int 2001;59:754–763.

6 Lang SM, Bergner A, Töpfer M, Schiffl H: Preservation of residual renal function in dialysis patients: effects of dialysis-technique-related factors. Perit Dial Int 2001;21:52–57.

7 Friedman AN, Fadem SZ: Reassessment of albumin as a nutritional marker in kidney disease. J Am Soc Nephrol 2010;21:223–230.

8 Steinman TI: Serum albumin: its significance in patients with ESRD. Semin Dial 2000;13:404–408.

9 Mehrotra R, Duong U, Jiwakanon S, Kovesdy CP, Moran J, Kopple JD, Kalantar-Zadeh K: Serum albumin as a predictor of mortality in peritoneal dialysis: comparisons with hemodialysis. Am J Kidney Dis 2011;58:418–428.

10 Hiramatsu M: How to improve survival in geriatric peritoneal dialysis patients. Perit Dial Int 2007;27:S185–S189.

11 Sueyoshi K, Inoue T, Kojima E, Sato T, Tsuda M, Kikuta T, Watanabe Y, Takane H, Takenaka T, Suzuki H: Clinical presentation in patients more than 80 years of age at the start of peritoneal dialysis. Adv Perit Dial 2011;27:71–76.

12 Suzuki H, Inoue T, Watanabe Y, Kikuta T, Sato T, Tsuda M: Survival of patients over 75 years of age on peritoneal dialysis therapy. Adv Perit Dial 2010;26:61–66.

13 Teitelbaum I: Peritoneal dialysis is appropriate for elderly patients. Contrib Nephrol. Basel, Karger, 2006, vol 150, pp 240–246.

14 Hiramatsu M: Improving outcome in geriatric dialysis patients. Perit Dial Int 2003;23:S84–S89.

15 Harris SA, Lamping DL, Brown EA, Constantinovici N: Clinical outcomes and quality of life in elderly patients on peritoneal dialysis versus hemodialysis. Perit Dial Int 2002;22:463–470.

16 Dombros NV: CAPD vs. hemodialysis in the elderly. Perit Dial 1988:291–296.

17 Brown EA: Peritoneal dialysis versus hemodialysis in the elderly. Perit Dial Int 1999;19:311–312.

18 Ismail N, Hakim RM, Oreopoulos DG, Patrikarea A: Renal replacement therapies in the elderly. 1. Hemodialysis and chronic peritoneal dialysis. Am J Kidney Dis 1993;22:759–782.

Makoto Hiramatsu, MD, PhD
Department of Nephrology, Okayama Saiseikai General Hospital
1-17-18 Ifuku-cho, Kita-ku
Okayama City, Okayama 700-8511 (Japan)
Tel. +81 86 252 2211, E-Mail m-hirama@saiseidr.jp

Hiramatsu · Ishida · Tonozuka · Mikami · Yamanari · Momoki · Onishi · Maruyama

Peritoneal Dialysis

Suzuki H (ed): Home Dialysis in Japan.
Contrib Nephrol. Basel, Karger, 2012, vol 177, pp 57–63

Maintenance of Continuous Ambulatory Peritoneal Dialysis in Elderly Patients

Mari Ishida

Kitasaito Hospital, Internal Medicine, Asahikawa City, Hokkaido, Japan

Abstract

In Japan, peritoneal dialysis (PD) remains the principal modality of home dialysis for the elderly although PD patients accounted for only 3.3% (n = 9,728) of the overall dialysis patient population. One of the preventing factors for introduction of PD in elderly patients is the Japanese public nursing care system. Besides, difficulties in the continuation of dialysis therapy will arise because of the progression of dementia as well as the decline in muscular strength, vigor, and physical strength of patients. In spite of these difficulties, some local dialysis centers tried to maintain and manage elderly dialysis patients at home by utilizing diverse social resources, in addition to obtaining the cooperation of caregivers such as family members. In our hospital, approximately 40% of patients who started dialysis therapy have selected PD. To support patients on PD, several special forms of care are prepared: utilization of visiting nurse care or home-visit nursing care services, supply of information on renal failure and education to home-care support providers and welfare service facility staff members. In addition, modulation of PD therapy such as automated PD and hemodialysis and PD in combination is also properly prepared. Lastly, the organization of a team, including physicians, nurses, social workers and dietitians, and the construction of a centralized patient information management system are important for elderly patients who need dialysis therapy.

Dialysis modalities are currently available for treating patients at home and are designated as home hemodialysis (HHD) and home peritoneal dialysis (PD), respectively. For HHD, regulations in Japan require the patient to have a caregiver at home and that the patient is able to perform needle insertions by him/herself. HHD is currently not indicated in elderly patients and patients with dementia. In fact, there are only 279 patients currently on HHD in Japan [1].

Thus, PD remains the principal modality of home dialysis for the elderly. According to a report that was released at the end of 2010 [1] by the Japanese

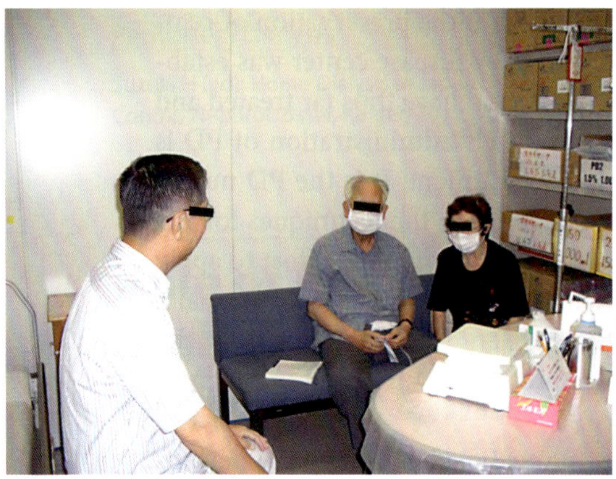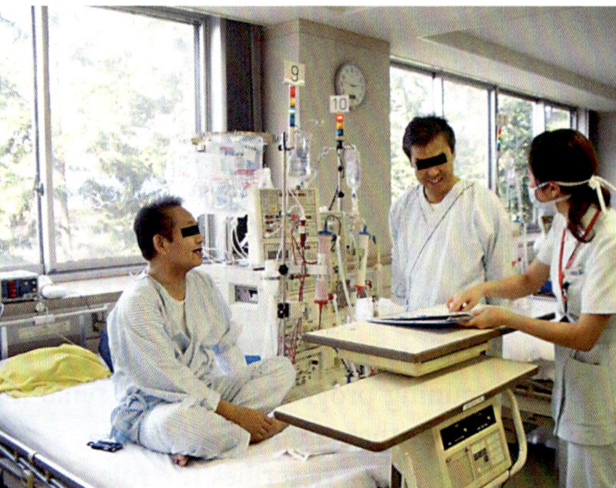

Fig. 1. Patient consultation (see text).

in consideration of their condition. Moreover, prepare explanations for family members who support patients so patients will not feel uneasy and alone.

(4) Give explanations that match the 'patient's level' clinically and psychologically. In particular, providing psychological support is an important role of nurses so that patients can accept RRT based on their emotional state at the time of the decision to introduce PD. The 'patient's level' indicates the point on the path toward reaching the final goal of 'acceptance of RRT'.

Usually, most patients follow a similar path that includes the following processes although the length of time to complete the process varies. It begins with 'shock', followed by 'distrust', 'denial', then 'anxiety and nervousness'. Sometimes there is 'depressed mood'. Finally, patients recognize that they must accept their need for some form of RRT. However, patients always have feelings that include both acceptance and refusal of dialysis, but the reality is the need for dialysis and in most cases acceptance is attained. The family as well as the nurse should display an understanding of such destructive emotions.

Nursing in PD Introduction Period

From the Decision of Introduction of PD to Tenckho® Catheter Insertion
Educational Goal. The patient should: (1) Understand the necessity of PD therapy and self-care. (2) Decide upon the brand of PD system he or she prefers (Terumo, Baxter, Fresenius, JMS, and others).

Instructional Content. (1) Basic information on PD: its principles and methods. (2) Practice of PD: common steps and equipment. (3) Characteristics of PD; advantages and disadvantages. (4) Gross outline of surgical techniques in Tenckhoff® catheter insertion (characteristics of Tenckhoff® catheter/

conditioning of catheter). (5) Explanation of PD systems and characteristics of each brand. (6) After patient decides on what PD system will be used, an explanation of the parts of that system should be given according to the brand. (7) Brief overview of daily self-care.

After Tenckhoff® Catheter Is Inserted: Introduction Period of Actual PD
Educational Goal. The patient should: (1) Understand the procedure necessary for self-administration of PD for home care and acquire the skills to perform the procedure. (2) Acquire knowledge of how to exchange bags with sterile technique. (3) Understand about peritonitis.

Instructional Content. (1) Necessity for and method of hand washing. (2) Bag exchange procedures. (3) Teaching the patient to record notes himself or herself. (4) Normal/abnormal findings of peritoneal dialysate. (5) Basic knowledge of PD-associated peritonitis. (6) Methodology for checking vital signs. (7) Body weight/blood pressure measurement. (8) Necessity and importance of fluid management, such as checking dialysate weight, body weight, urinary volume and water intake. (9) Methods for management of exit site; typical signs of tunnel infections. (10) Open shower bath method/bathing method for public baths and hot springs.

Before Leaving the Hospital
Educational Goal. The patient should: (1) Acquire the knowledge necessary for home care. (2) Gain confidence for self-administration and practice each step until it becomes automatic (bag exchange procedures, exit-site management, shower bathing method). (3) Understand and evaluate normal/abnormal conditions of the dialysate, exit site, and vital signs. (4) Independently conform to the treatment schedule.

Instructional Content. (1) Social security system. (2) Help patient prepare necessary supplies for PD in both the home and workplace (school). (3) Help patient determine a location for bag exchange procedures in home and workplace (school). (4) Schedule for bag exchange. (5) Diet therapy after introduction of PD. (6) Management of the delivery system for equipment. (7) Everyday life and social life. (8) Periodical outpatient consultation.

Important Nursing Issues during This Period
(1) Even when patients choose to undergo PD and have received dialysis, they cannot easily escape from anxiety and regret. Therefore, nurses must provide them with the knowledge and skills necessary for self-administration of PD while they support patients by displaying empathy, drawing out their conflicts and listening to them so that they are better able to accept dialysis.

(2) There are individual differences among patients in the level of understanding of information given and technical guidance on PD. Therefore, nurses must provide explanations repeatedly, such as reiterating issues such as 'why dialysis is necessary' and 'why this procedure is used'.

(3) Nurses can support patients so that they can accept their own anxieties about surgery and a change in body image after the operation.

(4) In the PD introduction period, helping patients understand and imagine how PD, which will begin in the future, will be added to the patient's life can lead to the further acceptance of dialysis and the motivation to perform it. Therefore, nurses must have a good rapport with patients so that they can express anxiety over their social life to nurses. Nurses should recognize patients' anxieties and provide the knowledge and information to decrease this anxiety. It is important to support such patients so that they can solve their problems in an effective and unique way particularly suited to their own situation.

Nursing in the Peritoneal Dialysis Maintenance Period

Educational Goal. The patient should: Plan maintenance of their general condition and improve quality of life by self-care.

Instructional Content. At this point, instruction is combined with observation of and interaction with patients during visits to the dialysis center. (1) Assist physicians with physical examinations. At this time, observe the patient's general condition and ask the patient about his or her general condition, such as changes in body weight, dialysate volume, blood pressure at home, etc. This will provide clues as to what further education is needed. (2) Check patient's notes made since previous visit. (3) Check laboratory data. (4) Observe exit site and verify care of the site. (5) Confirm the patient's understanding of bag exchange procedures. (6) Explain rationale for various examinations (blood tests/cell count in dialysate/ urinalysis/thoracoabdominal X-ray/electrocardiography, etc.). (7) Provide counseling/instruction in accordance with patient's condition. (8) Check on supplies, adjustment of equipment and dialysate. (9) Explain about periodic connection tube replacement. (10) Provide support in the transition period from PD to HD, home HD and renal transplantation, as may be necessary.

Important Nursing Issues during This Period
(1) As patients only visit the hospital once a month, it is important for nurses to be in contact with patients in order to understand their living conditions, to provide appropriate instructions and advice, and perform counseling on issues that have arisen.

(2) Nurses tend to feel relieved when a patient performs sufficient self-administration of PD without serious difficulties. However, it is important to confirm the bag exchange operation using a checklist and repeatedly review instructions, giving plenty of feedback. A flow chart should be provided for emergency and abnormal situations.

(3) As use of PD can be considered a transition period prior to the need for HD and other forms of RRT, nurses must again provide information on various

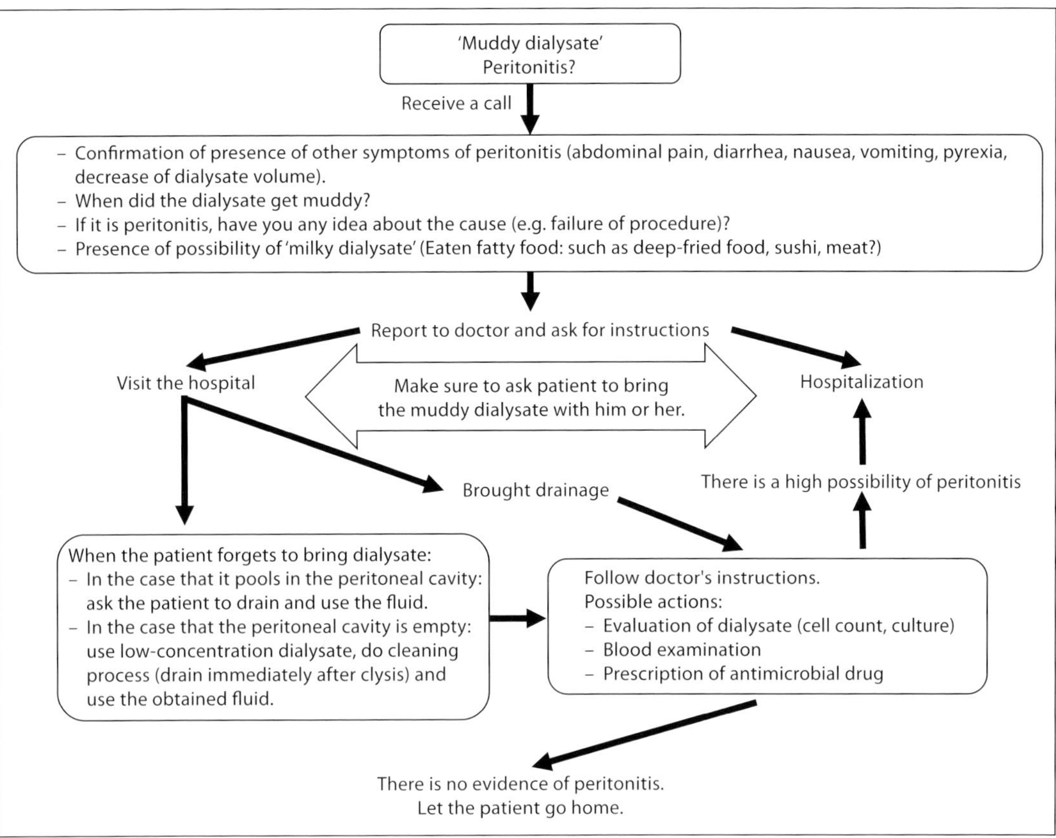

Fig. 2. Flow chart for peritonitis.

forms of RRTs and to plan with their patients how they can achieve a positive image of life after the transition period.

(4) The nursing care plan should be continuously revised based on changes in the patient's physical and psychological condition. Included in this care plan should be a plan for individualized education based on observations made during this period.

In our hospital, the Nephrology and Dialysis Unit has also established a backup system for not only PD patients but also for many home HD patients. A full-time renal consultation service, including cooperation between Nephrology and other departments, is recommended. Moreover, guidelines and protocols for management of common dialysis-related complications (PD-associated peritonitis, exit-site infection, clogged PD catheter, etc.) should be made available to the all staff in Nephrology and the Dialysis Unit. As the occasion demands, we should provide supportive and temporal HD with a double-lumen catheter without undue delay. For instance, the flow chart for peritonitis is shown in figure 2.

Conclusion

In this chapter, the authors described nursing care with a strong emphasis on education for PD patients from the introduction to the maintenance period. Shigekazu Haruki (psycho-nephrologist in Japan) said, 'I believe healing their "psychological wound" will be our task prior to "education". We cannot go forward without it'. We believe that displaying empathy to a patient, that is, putting ourselves in the position of the patient, and fostering an ongoing interaction between ourselves and the patient will build a confident relationship between the nurse and patient and provide the patient with good nursing care.

References

1 Chaudhary K, Sangha H, Khanna R: Peritoneal dialysis first: rationale. Clin J Am Soc Nephrol 2011;6:447–456.
2 Kong IL, Yip IL, Mok GW, Chan SY, Tang CM, Wong SW, et al: Setting up a continuous ambulatory peritoneal dialysis training program. Perit Dial Int 2003;23(suppl 2): S178–S182.
3 Sadala ML, Miranda MG, Lorencon M, de Campos Pereira EP: Nurse-patient communication while performing home dialysis: the patients' perceptions. J Ren Care 2010;36: 34–40.

Hiromichi Suzuki, MD, PhD
38 Morohongo, Moroyama-machi, Iruma-gun
Saitama 350-0495 (Japan)
Tel. +81 49 2761612
E-Mail iromichi@saitama-med.ac.jp

Suzuki H (ed): Home Dialysis in Japan.
Contrib Nephrol. Basel, Karger, 2012, vol 177, pp 71–83

Combination Therapy with Hemodialysis and Peritoneal Dialysis

Hiromichi Suzuki · Hitosi Hoshi · Tsutomu Inoue · Tomohiro Kikuta · Masahiro Tsuda · Tsuneo Takenaka

Department of Nephrology, Saitama Medical University, Saitama, Japan

Abstract

Both continuous ambulatory peritoneal dialysis (CAPD) and hemodialysis (HD) have their advantages regarding the treatment of patients with renal failure. In CAPD, solute removal is sometimes insufficient in patients who have a relatively large muscle mass that produces high levels of creatinine. To compensate for this deficiency, frequent exchanges and large peritoneal dialysate volumes are required. Alternatively, CAPD and HD as a combined modality of treatment for patients needing dialysis therapy has been proposed. Our experiences with three groups of patients are described. First, in 2003, 7 cases (6 males and 1 female; average age 54.3 ± 4.5 years; mean duration of CAPD therapy 4.3 ± 1.1 years; average weekly creatinine clearance (WCC) was 45.2 ± 1.7 l/1.73 m^2) were treated with once-a-week HD therapy (3.5 h; 200 ml/h). Addition of once-a-week HD therapy improved WCC to 66 ± 7.1 liters/1.73 m^2. This improvement was due not only to the addition of HD therapy but also to an increase in creatinine clearance for 3 consecutive days after the completion of once-a-week HD therapy. Both creatinine clearance and ultrafiltration were significantly increased. Other clinical parameters such as blood pressure control, weight control, and dosage of erythropoietin were significantly improved after introducing this therapy. Second, we followed 9 CAPD patients who underwent an additional weekly HD for more than 3 years. Similar improvements were obtained in this long-term study as seen in the short-term study. Besides, the incidence of peritonitis decreased dramatically from 0.13 to 0.09 episodes/patient-year (p < 0.05) during the 3-year study. These data suggest that the combined use of CAPD and HD improves solute clearance in CAPD patients who are insufficiently dialyzed. Third, based on these data, we examined the efficacy of an early start of combination therapy and found that it stabilized dialysis therapy and prolonged the duration of CAPD. Combined with several of the previous several reports and our present experience, it is suggested that an early start of HD therapy will prolong the survival rate in patients on CAPD with physically stable conditions.

Although continuous ambulatory peritoneal dialysis (CAPD) has been advocated as an initial therapy [1], an increase in patients choosing CAPD has only recently been recorded [2]. The major reason for patients with end-stage renal disease (ESRD) not selecting CAPD as an initial modality of dialysis therapy is that if CAPD therapy fails for whatever reason (usually peritonitis, inadequate dialysis, or patient-related factors), then a switch from CAPD to hemodialysis (HD) would need to be considered. One problem with this approach is that CAPD patients are transferred to HD in spite of retaining peritoneal function. Among the factors considered for discontinuing CAPD, peritoneal transport status, which may be associated with adverse clinical outcome [3], is of utmost importance. Moreover, the association of peritoneal transport status and weekly creatinine clearance (WCC) needs to be monitored [4, 5]. Guidelines on targets for solute clearance have now been published, the most prominent of which is the National Kidney Foundation-Dialysis Outcomes Quality Initiative (NKF-DOQI) guidelines [6]. The NKF-DOQI targets a WCC of >60 liters/1.73 m^2. Adequate WCC can be achieved by several methods. One method is an automated PD (APD), although no decisive data are available for the effects of increasing usage on patients' outcomes. Since one HD session is equivalent to 2–3 days of CAPD in terms of creatinine clearance (CrCl), the addition of HD to CAPD patients who do not achieve the WCC targets would be an alternative [7, 8]. Considerable obstacles exist for this approach that is almost entirely non-medical, such as physician biases, conservative policies and so on. 'PD + HD combination therapy' was the name proposed in 1996 by Kimura and Watanabe in Japan. In 2003, an ad-hoc committee of the International Society of Peritoneal Dialysis labeled this therapy as 'complementary dialysis therapy'. McIntyre [9] proposed the name 'bimodal dialysis'. Ten years ago, there were only a few studies in this field published in English [7, 10]. Recently however, a number of studies have been reported in English [11–16]. In this report the aim is to describe three studies [12, 17] conducted in The Kidney Disease Center in Saitama Medical University Hospital since 1998 and to discuss the feasibility of these approaches in treating ESRD.

Regular Treatment Modality in the Kidney Center in Saitama Medical University

More than 60% of patients were treated with a standard CAPD regimen that consisted of four daily exchanges of 1.5 or 2 liters of dialysate, while other patients used two to three daily exchanges of dialysate. The strength of the bags was individualized to maintain the desired weight. Dwell times were also individualized to maximize overall ultrafiltration volumes. During the study, all subjects were asked to maintain their customary dietary and dialysis regimen.

Mean daily dietary intake was recorded from individual 24-hour food records during a 3-day period at the start of the study. All subjects consumed between 0.8 and 1.0 g of protein/kg/day and their energy intake exceeded 25 kcal/kg/day. Salt intake was restricted to <9 g/day.

Weekly assessments of residual renal function (liters/week) of the subjects were estimated from their mean renal creatinine and urea clearances determined daily from their 24-hour urine collections. WCCs were calculated from 24-hour spent dialysates. Both serum and peritoneal creatinine concentrations were measured. CrCl by HD was calculated using the following formula: creatinine concentration × (dialysate flow × duration of dialysis + removal fluid). All subjects used the same dialyzer for 3.5 h. CrCl by HD was found to be 2,000–2,400 mg.

Patient Monitoring

Patients underwent the standard monthly assessment of biochemical and hematological indices. Data were recorded on pre- and post-HD blood pressure, antihypertensive medication use, response to epoetin and doses, calcium/phosphate control, and hyperparathyroidism. If a subject's systolic blood pressure (SBP) exceeded 140 mm Hg or diastolic blood pressure (DBP) exceeded 90 mm Hg, antihypertensive therapy was initiated. The selection of antihypertensive agent depended on the physicians' preference.

During the study period, subjects were treated with recombinant human erythropoietin (rHuEPO) as necessary and their hemoglobin levels were maintained between 10 and 11 g/dl. Subjects were given oral iron supplementation if they were diagnosed with iron deficiency.

Subjects with parathyroid hormone levels >200 pg/ml were treated with $1,25(OH)_2D_3$ and $CaCO_3$ supplements, while patients with levels <70 pg/ml were treated with $CaCO_3$ to reduce the degree of hyperphosphatemia. Doses were adjusted based on serum levels of calcium and phosphate. Lipid-lowering drugs, primarily statin derivatives, were administered if serum cholesterol levels exceeded 240 mg/dl. The following parameters were measured: blood urea nitrogen, serum creatinine, electrolytes, calcium, phosphate, and alkaline phosphatase, hemoglobin, and hematocrit. Parathyroid hormone levels (intact molecule assay) and serum cholesterol were also measured.

Informed consent was obtained. Baseline data, including age, sex, underlying renal disease, CAPD regimen, duration of CAPD, dialysis regimen, and past history of peritonitis were obtained. The following types of patients were excluded: (1) those unlikely to survive for 6 months; (2) those planning to have an elective living donor transplant, or (3) those transferring to another renal center within 6 months.

Table 1. Characteristics of patients

Initial	Age (years)	Sex	Underlying disease	Duration of CAOD (years)	Past history of peritonitis
KH	47	M	CGN	2.5	0
AS	63	M	Bechet	4.2	1
HS	56	M	CGN	3.1	0
HI	45	F	CGN	5.2	0
IM	56	M	CGN	4.2	1
TT	67	M	NS	4.5	1
YM	39	M	CGN	4.1	1
	54 ± 4			4.3 ± 1.1	

M = Male; F = female; CGN = chronic glomerular disease; NS = nephrosclerosis.

Statistical Analysis

All data are presented as the mean ± SD. Comparisons between starting values and values obtained at one of the other time points of the study were made using Student's t test, with a p value of <0.05 indicating statistical significance. Regression analyses were performed to compare the levels of serum albumin and hemoglobin, with the WCC being the independent variable.

Short-Term Effects of Combination Therapy

Patient Selection. Seven CAPD patients, who were admitted to the Kidney Disease Center of Saitama Medical University Hospital between 1998 and 2001, were eligible for the study.

Characteristics of Patients (table 1). Age, sex, serum creatinine, duration of CAPD and past history of peritonitis are described in table 1. Only 1 of the 7 patients was a female. The duration of CAPD was less than 5 years. Underlying renal disease was predominantly chronic glomerular nephritis. The frequency of peritonitis was less than twice in all patients. The urine volumes of all patients were <100 ml/day.

Effects of Add-On HD Therapy on Peritoneal CrCl. Add-on HD therapy increased weekly peritoneal CrCl from 45 ± 1.7 to 48 ± 2.1 liters (p < 0.05). Then 48 liters were added by 24 liters of CrCl by HD, reaching a total WCC >60 liters (fig. 1).

Effects of Add-On HD Therapy on Drain Volume. The daily drain volume increased from 890 ± 75 to 1,150 ± 90 ml/day after addition of once-a-week HD (p < 0.01) (fig. 2).

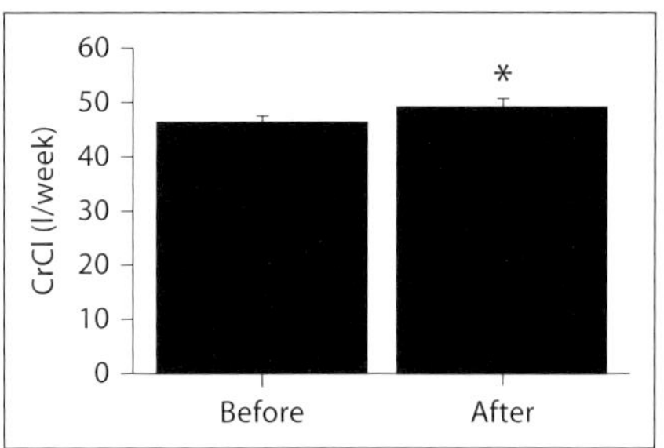

Fig. 1. Effects of add-on HD therapy on peritoneal CrCl. Add-on HD therapy increased weekly peritoneal CrCl from 45 + 1.7 to 48 + 2.1 liters (*p < 0.05).

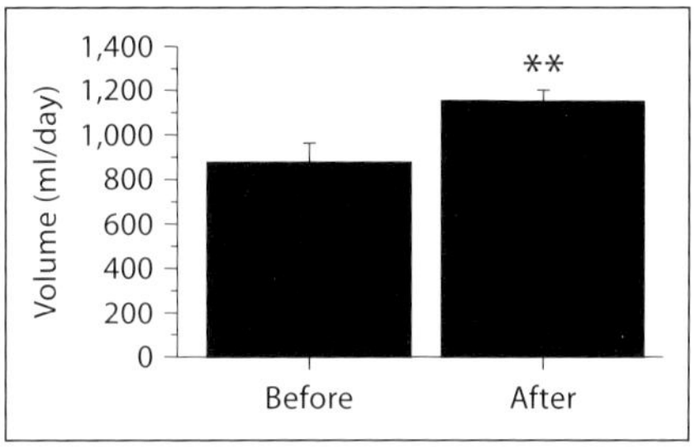

Fig. 2. Effects of add-on HD therapy on drain volume. The daily drain volume increased after addition of once-a-week HD (**p < 0.01).

Effects of Add-On HD Therapy on Serum Creatinine. The levels of serum creatinine decreased from 12.3 ± 0.9 to 11.0 ± 0.6 mg/dl by addition of once-a-week HD (p < 0.05).

Long-Term Effects of Combination Therapy

Patients. Nine CAPD patients, who were admitted to the Kidney Disease Center of Saitama Medical University Hospital between 1998 and 2005, were enrolled in this study.

Subjects' Characteristics. The subjects' mean age, sex ratio, mean duration of CAPD, underlying renal disease and incidence of peritonitis at the beginning of the study were as follows: 58 ± 7 years; 8/1 male/female; 3.6 ± 0.2 years; chronic glomerulonephritis 6, nephrosclerosis 1, diabetes mellitus 1, and Beçhet's disease 1. All subjects survived beyond the 3 years of the study and none were transferred to HD alone. Parathyroidectomy was performed in 1 patient because he had a serum PTH value of >1,000 mg/dl; this subject was subsequently found to have had multiple parathyroidal adenomas.

Follow-Up Data of SBP and DBP, Serum Creatinine, Blood Urea Nitrogen, Hemoglobin, Potassium, Calcium, Phosphate and Total Cholesterol (table 2). There were no differences in DBP, serum creatinine, blood urea nitrogen, potassium, calcium, phosphate, and total cholesterol during the 3 years of the study

Table 2. Follow-up laboratory and dialysis data during 3 years

	0	1	2	3
Systolic blood pressure (mm Hg)	140.8	135.3	131.7*	132.1*
	4.7	3.6	3.0	5.5
Diastolic blood pressure (mm Hg)	72.3	69.5	70.3	70.5
	3.8	4.1	3.6	3.6
Serum creatinine (mg/dl)	13.5	13.6	12.7	12.9
	0.8	0.5	1.0	0.9
Blood urea nitrogen (mg/dl)	76.4	70.7	63.8	67.6
	7.8	3.0	4.5	2.8
Serum albumin (g/dl)	3.66	3.78	4.12*	4.03*
	0.25	0.25	0.18	0.2
Serum calcium (mg/dl)	8.49	9.05	9.72	8.84
	0.46	0.55	0.25	0.51
Serum phosphate (mg/dl)	7.2	7.6	6.5	7.5
	0.7	0.6	0.7	0.7
Serum potassium (mEq/l)	4.8	4.7	4.3	4.5
	0.3	0.3	0.2	0.3
Total cholesterol (mg/dl)	164.6	162.0	146.2	158.0
	7.6	7.6	9.3	9.5
Drain volume (ml/day)	716	744*	916*	916*
	125	131	76	121
Weekly creatinine clearance (l/week)	47.6	60.5*	62.8*	61.7*
	2.2	3.1	4.2	4.7
Hemoglobin (g/dl)	7.7	8.2	8.6*	8.7*
	0.6	0.3	0.4	0.5
Intact PTH (mg/dl)	386	388	512	366
	124	138	266	299

Values are expressed as mean in the upper column and standard deviation in the lower column. *indicates a significance at level of $P < 0.05$ compared to the value at year 0.

compared to starting values. On the other hand, SBP and serum albumin and hemoglobin levels gradually increased, and the values achieved significance at years 2 and 3 ($p < 0.05$).

Changes in WCC and Drain Volume (fig. 3, 4). Both WCC and drain volume increased by year 1 ($p < 0.05$), and remained elevated over the subsequent 2 years.

Correlation between WCC and Serum Albumin and Hemoglobin Levels (fig. 5). There was a significant correlation ($p < 0.05$) between CrCl and serum albumin levels (fig. 3), but not between CrCl and hemoglobin and SBP.

Incidence of Peritonitis. The incidence of peritonitis decreased dramatically from 0.13 to 0.09 episodes/patient-year ($p < 0.05$) during the 3-year study.

Dose of rHuEPO. Before the start of add-on HD therapy, the average required dose of rHuEPO was 5,500 ± 600 IU/month. However, since hemoglobin levels

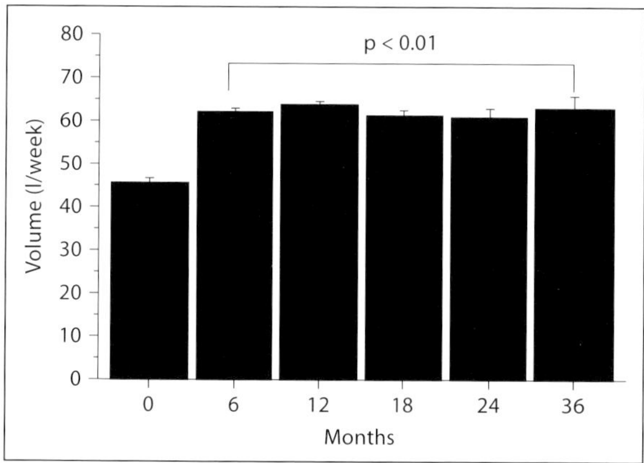

Fig. 3. Changes in WCC during the study period paralleled the changes in drain volume. p < 0.01 compared with values at month 0.

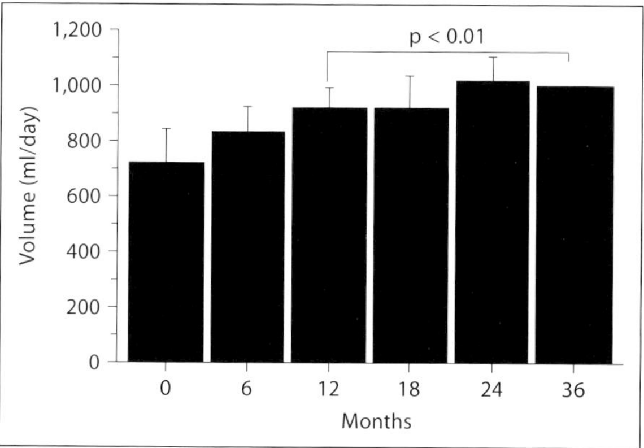

Fig. 4. Changes in drain volume during the 3-year follow-up. Drain volume gradually increased toward the end of the first year and reached the significant level, then it was stabilized during the next 2 years. p < 0.01 compared with values at month 0.

increased gradually in response to our treatment regimen, subjects required reduced doses of rHuEPO (5,000 ± 600 IU).

Antihypertensive Medication. The blood pressures of 5 subjects decreased after the start of add-on HD therapy and their antihypertensive treatment regimens were reduced.

Effects of Early Start of Combination Therapy

Patients. Ten CAPD patients who started combination therapy within 1 year after the initiation of CAPD were enrolled in this study.

these changes to GPs. Specialists make reservations for medical examinations after 3–18 months, depending on patient renal function. When GPs cooperate with specialists from the early stage of CKD, they can give medical care as chief physicians until patients enter the advanced stage, which is defined by a serum creatinine (Cr) concentration of >5.0 mg/dl, except in the elderly, those with severe overhydration, and those with severe hyperkalemia.

Education Program for CKD Patients

When conducting an education program for CKD patients, it is important to first build mutual trust by continuing the periodic cooperation through cooperation tools, which are easy to use and will not frustrate patients.

Clinical Pathways Shared with GPs
The KDTS has developed a cooperation program for CKD involving the following: three parties (the patient, the GP, and a specialist), a clinical pathway, and three copies of a medical report. For patients introduced by a GP, specialists examine CKD and CVD in detail, and the contents of prescriptions, results of laboratory testing, and other matters that require attention are addressed in the report. The GPs continue issuing the prescription advised by the specialists and perform appropriate laboratory tests at specified intervals. Because reports containing patient medical records recorded by the GP and specialist are included in the cooperation pathway, patients can confirm the exchange of medical information via the pathway. This improves the quality of healthcare services, builds mutual trust, and overcomes progression of CKD through a three-way patient-centered periodic cooperation program.

Blood Pressure, Pulse Rate, Blood Glucose, Body Weight, and Data from Patient Diaries
Blood pressure, pulse rate, blood glucose, and body weight fluctuate over the course of CKD. When patients do not measure these parameters at home, it becomes difficult to delay the progression of CKD despite appropriate lifestyle, diet, and pharmacotherapy.

Pamphlet on Diabetes, Hypertension, and CKD
It is important to educate CKD patients through a pamphlet with details on CKD and RRTs.

Predialysis Education for Patients
Many patients have trouble in clearly understanding CKD, even after reading a pamphlet about their condition. Therefore, it is essential that healthcare workers clearly inform patients about CKD.

Public Lectures on CKD
CKD is a serious public health problem. The International Kidney Evaluation Association of Japan introduced the Kidney Early Evaluation Program, developed by the National Kidney Foundation, and found that approximately 25% of participants with risk factors had CKD [3]. Although there are many CKD patients in Japan and only a few institutions that can perform all RRTs, we send information according to the units in individual areas that can perform all RRTs. Furthermore, it is important that patients choose the RRT that is best for them. Therefore, hosting public lectures that can forge strong bonds with participants is desirable.

Examples of Public Lectures
The theme of the fifth KDTS public lecture series, supported by the Tokyo Metropolitan Government and conducted on December 11, 2010, was proper acquaintance with CKD. Over 400 people attended from Saitama, Kanagawa, Gunma, Yamanashi, and Chiba, in addition to the Tokyo area. Many patients gained valuable information on CKD as the lecture covered topics including CKD, diet therapy, living guidance, pharmacotherapy, RTx, HHD, and PD.

Display Booths Relating to CKD Therapy with Public Lectures
The KDTS hosted display booths on the theme 'Measures of CKD' after the above-mentioned lectures to deepen participant understanding of CKD. Other booth themes included medical cooperation, measurement of blood pressure and blood sugar, walking therapy, diet therapy, pharmacotherapy, RTx, conventional HD and HHD, buttonhole insertion, and PD. Unlike the lectures, display booths allowed the participants to question healthcare workers directly. Many participants also watched and experienced instruments in use. The exhibition helped participants who were nervous about asking questions during the lecture to understand RRTs correctly.

PD Promotion Program

The KDTS conducts a PD promotion program by issuing pamphlets, providing predialysis education, and giving public lectures.

Importance of Maintaining Residual Renal Function
We treated CKD patients in the predialysis stage to maintain residual renal function (RRF). A close relationship between RRF and survival after dialysis is initiated has been reported [4]. In addition, it has been reported that patients who are transferred from PD to HD have better overall survival than those who start and remain on HD [5]. Furthermore, PD patients are associated with improved survival for up to 48 months compared with HD patients [6].

Therefore, it is important to continue treatment to maintain RRF after starting PD.

Intermittent Ambulatory Peritoneal Dialysis and Intermittent Automated Peritoneal Dialysis

PD is thought to be required daily for patients with end-stage CKD. Many PD patients report that performing PD bag exchanges daily are stressful [7]. However, we report that intermittent PD prescription, namely intermittent ambulatory peritoneal dialysis or intermittent automated peritoneal dialysis, which is defined as PD prescription with more than 1 PD rest day (PD holiday) during the week, is feasible when a patient's RRF is relatively stable [8, 9]. However, a few patients with intermittent PD prescription, who were unable to accept water restrictions, were admitted to the hospital due to severe overhydration. To perform adequate ultrafiltration, we introduced the concept of 'danger weight' [10]. When a patient's body weight exceeds the danger weight, the patient must restrict water intake and undergo ultrafiltration by increasing dialysate glucose concentration or by canceling their PD holiday to normalize their fluid volume at home. Because intermittent PD prescription is attractive for patients as a means of obtaining PD holidays, many patients in our hospital have selected the intermittent PD prescription. Some patients with good control of blood pressure, glucose, lipids, uric acid, and anemia have been on an intermittent PD prescription without any clinical problem for over 10 years. It is important to maintain an adequate dialysis index with a decrease in RRT for continuing intermittent PD over a long period; formulas for peritoneal and renal Kt/V and peritoneal and renal Cr clearance in intermittent PD are shown in table 1.

Intracorporeal Ultrafiltration Method

The extracorporeal ultrafiltration method (ECUM) [11] has been used to treat severe overhydration in CKD patients. Because a PD solution containing icodextrin was introduced to manage sustained ultrafiltration over a long dwelling time [12], PD with icodextrin dialysate can be used to manage patients who need periodic ultrafiltration. We report that CKD patients with overhydration were successfully managed using the intracorporeal ultrafiltration method (ICUM), which consists of 1,500 ml icodextrin dialysate for a single overnight exchange (10 h) 5 times per week with a restricted water intake of 500 ml per day [13].

ICUM can be started in the outpatient department. After a PD catheter is inserted, the patient receives PD education and sham training for bag exchange. When dialysis is initiated, the patient performs a real bag exchange once a day for several days in the outpatient department. The patient undergoes ICUM with a PD holiday at home after it is confirmed that there are no problems with bag exchanges. One patient with good control of blood pressure, glucose,

Table 1. Formulas for peritoneal and renal Kt/V and peritoneal and renal creatinine clearance in intermittent PD

$$\text{Peritoneal Kt/V urea (/week)} = \frac{\dfrac{\text{Dialysate UN}}{\text{Serum UN}} \times \dfrac{\text{Drain volume}}{1{,}000}}{\text{Body weight} \times 0.58} \times \text{PD days/week}$$

$$\text{Renal Kt/V urea (/week)} = \frac{\dfrac{\text{Urinary UN}}{\text{Serum UN}} + \dfrac{\text{Urine volume}}{1{,}000}}{\text{Body weight} \times 0.58} \times 7$$

$$\text{Peritoneal clearance (l/week/1.73 m}^2) = \frac{\text{Dialysate Cr}}{\text{Serum Cr}} \times \frac{\text{Drain volume}}{1{,}000} \times \text{PD days/week} \times \frac{1.73}{\text{Body surface area}}$$

$$\text{Renal clearance (l/week/1.73 m}^2) = \frac{\dfrac{\text{Urinary Cr}}{\text{Serum Cr}} + \dfrac{\text{Urinary UN}}{\text{Serum UN}}}{2} \times \frac{\text{Urine volume}}{1{,}000} \times 7 \times \frac{1.73}{\text{Body surface area}}$$

Units are: UN (urea nitrogen), mg/dl; Cr (creatinine), mg/dl; Drain volume, urine volume, ml/day; Body weight, kg, and Body surface area, m^2.

lipids, uric acid, and anemia was on ICUM for over 4 years, without any clinical problems.

Venovenous Extracorporeal Ultrafiltration Method
We retrospectively analyzed the effects of ECUM via peripheral veins (venovenous ECUM; VVECUM) in PD patients with excessive body fluid retention and decreasing RRF. Two veins, either in the forearm or upper arm, are punctured using 16-gauge needles, and the blood flow rate is kept at 60–100 ml/min; treatment time is around 2 h. Based on the hydration status, we normalized the fluid volume in all patients by regulating the number of treatment days for individual patients. Treatment with PD alone was possible after fluid volume normalization by VVECUM in many patients for 4–6 months if they strictly adhered to water intake limitations. Furthermore, long-term (>42 months) PD therapy was successfully continued in a case with sufficient ultrafiltration volume by using PD and with good fluid intake control. Without VVECUM treatment, all cases would have been immediately transferred onto HD because of severe fluid retention. These results suggest that VVECUM treatment makes PD patients aware of HD, motivating them to continue PD (which is chosen by the patients themselves) and maintain strict fluid intake restrictions [14]. Because this method does not cause arteriovenous fistula (AVF), the heart is protected.

Care during the Maintenance Stage of Home Dialysis Treatment

Peritoneal dialysis (PD) comes in various safe and easy-to-operate treatments, including automated peritoneal dialysis (APD), which has recently been promoted on a global scale, as well as the most popular CAPD. Treatment can be chosen according to lifestyle. The goal of the nursing is to give instructions based on the results of biochemical examination and peritoneal function test, in order to choose the appropriate treatment. Disadvantages of CAPD are especially underdialysis and overhydration, and must be avoided. Nutrition education regarding albumin and potassium loss and glucose absorption due to the use of PD fluid, which are unique to CAPD, education on prevention of peritonitis exit-site infection and peritoneal catheter care, which occur only in CAPD, instructions regarding bathing, and nursing from a certified nurse specialist are vital.

In order to continue HHD, the existence of a helper is the most important problem in nursing. The helpers of 66 patients with HHD were investigated. As a result, 59 helpers were female (52 ± 11 years old, range 28–80) and 7 were males (56 ± 10 years old, range 37–69). The combination in Japan that the husband is the HHD patient and the wife is the helper was found in 52 persons (79%), it was the mother in 6 persons (9.1%), the husband in 5 persons (7.6%), and the father and elder sister and younger brother in each 1 person respectively. It is an important problem that HHD continues in the future when the helper becomes older.

The goal of nursing in HHD during the maintenance stage is to support the patient so that dialysis therapy can be carried out properly and safely as a part of the patient's lifestyle, to quickly detect physiological abnormalities, and to prevent complications. Content and frequency of contact from HHD patients and the staff are shown in table 1. Regarding contact and inquiry, and materials for dialysis, most inquiries involved the physical condition of the patient, such as change in physical shape, external injury, and bone fracture, but there was only one emergency house visit within a year among 41 people under management. Clinical engineers handled equipment management. The most common inquiries concerned problems with the dialysis equipment and equipment trouble caused by operation and damaged machinery.

Gist of Care during Discontinuation of Home Dialysis Therapy

CAPD is discontinued in cases where insufficient peritoneal function occurs, intractability especially due to peritonitis caused by fungal infection [5, 6]. Special care must be taken when nursing, since removing the catheter immediately during the discontinuation period may result in encapsulated peritoneal sclerosis. HHD is discontinued in cases of complication requiring hospital

Table 1. Interconnection frequency between HHD patients and management facility (for 1 year in 41 patients, 2011)

Telephone interconnection			Home visit		
In the time	25–50 (48)/M	572/year	Urgent visit		1 fre/year
The time outside	2–24 (13)/M	149/year	Education visit	0–4 (2)/M	23 fre/year
			Periodic visit	3–20 (11)/M	129 fre/year

Item	From patient		From facility		Item	From patient	From facility
Material	96 (8)	4–12		3–	Education	15 (1.3)	0–3
Machine	109 (9)	1–15	17 (1.4)	0–5	Dosing and treatment	6 –	0–2
Communication query	298 (25)	15–35	89 (7.4)	3–15	Assistance	4 –	0–2
Consultation report	162 (14)	5–24			Inspection	57 (5)	0–11
Body condition	56 (5)	1–10		0–4	Machine repair	17 (1.4)	0–5
					Others	53 (44)	7–20
Total	721 (60.1)		95 (8)		Total	152 (13)	

fre = Frequency. Average frequency in 1 month is given in parentheses.

treatment, or when the helper is too old and can no longer care for the patient. Some patients still prefer home dialysis and switch to CAPD.

Conclusion

Although the utilization rate of CAPD and especially HHD (both home dialysis) is still low in Japan, measures to prevent complications unique to CAPD have been gradually put in place over the past 22 years. As a result, the possibility of a rapid increase in CAPD can be seen on the horizon. On the other hand, for HHD, the other home dialysis, the difficulty of a puncture can be overcome by creating a buttonhole and changing the 'puncture' to an 'insert'. It is likely that the home dialysis will gain popularity by developing equipment which is easy to operate, improving the support facilities, promoting nursing, and making full use of social resources such as home management services.

References

1 Just PM, de Charro FT, Tschosik EA, Noe LL, Bhattacharyya SK, Riella MC: Reibursement and economic factors influencing dialysis modality choice around the world. Nephrol Dial Transplant 2008;23:2365–2373.

2 The Statistical Survey Committee and the Statistical Analysis Subcommittee of JSDT: An overview of regular treatment in Japan (as of December 31, 2009). J Jpn Soc Dial Ther 2001;44:1–36.

3   Wong JHS, Pierratos A, Oreopoulos DG, Mohammad R, Benjamin-Wong F, Chan CT: The use of nocturnal home hemodialysis as salvage therapy for patients experiencing peritoneal dialysis failure. Perit Dial Int 2007; 27:669–674.

4   Kawanishi H, Hashimoto Y, Nakamoto H, Nakayama M, Tranaeus A: Combination therapy with peritoneal dialysis and hemodialysis. Perit Dial Int 2006;26:150–154.

5   Kawaguchi Y, Ishizaki T, Imada A, Oohira S, Kuriyama S, Nakamoto H, Nakamoto M, Hiramatsu M, Maeda K, Ota K, Study Group for Withdrawal from Peritoneal Dialysis: Nationwide survey in Japan. Perit Dial Int 2003;23(suppl 2):S175–S177.

6   Kawaguchi Y, Saito A, Kawanishi H, Nakayama M, Miyazaki M, Nakamoto H, Tranaeus A: Recommendation on the management of encapsulating peritoneal sclerosis in Japan 2005. Diagnosis, Predictive makers, treatment and preventive measures. Perit Dial Int 2005;25(suppl 4):S83–S95.

Dr. Akio Imada
3-4-14 Nishi-Yamamoto-cho
Yao City, Osaka 581-0868 (Japan)
Tel. +81 72 923 0490
E-Mail aimada@jshd.jp

Suzuki H (ed): Home Dialysis in Japan.
Contrib Nephrol. Basel, Karger, 2012, vol 177, pp 99–105

Perspectives on Home Hemodialysis in Japan

Kenji Maeda[a] · Shigeru Nakai[b]

[a]Daiko-Sunadabashi Clinic and [b]Division of Clinical Engineering Technology, Fujita Health University School of Health Sciences, Nagoya, Japan

Abstract

Home hemodialysis (HHD) started in Japan in 1969. It has been done in the largest number of patients with the purpose of better social reintegration, followed by patients for whom commuting to a hospital is geographically difficult. In a subanalysis of the JSDT patient registry, the survival rate at 9 years for male patients excluding those with diabetes was significantly better in HHD patients than in facility dialysis patients. This result was thought to indicate that HHD was superior treatment both medically and socially, but it has not increased greatly because of conditions that impede the implementation of HHD, such as finding a caregiver and the burden on the caregiver, as well as the burden of light, heat, and water costs. However, long-duration dialysis and frequent dialysis are done even in general dialysis treatment, and the number of HHD patients has increased recently because of some improvement in health insurance payments for HHD in 1998. The spread of HHD is essential also in the broad implementation of diversifying HD modalities, and maintaining an accurate registry of HHD patients, analyzing factors that affect survival rates with each modality, clarifying conditions for adequacy of dialysis, and clarifying which treatments are superior are important future issues for dialysis treatment.

Home hemodialysis (HHD) began at Nagoya University Branch Hospital in Japan in 1969. It was done with the Kill dialyzer, using a personal use dialysis solution delivery system for the home developed by a Japanese company. The service initially targeted patients with the ability to understand the process and who, as a rule, had one person to assist. HHD was judged to be possible based on an investigation of the housing situation, economic status, possibility of social reintegration, and geographic conditions. The basic conditions were dialysis for 8 h/session, 3 sessions/week. A 24-hour on-call system was established.

especially to improving the results of HHD treatment. A search for factors that contribute to the adequacy of hemodialysis revealed that various hemodialysis methods have been evaluated based on quantitative analysis of guanidine compounds [8], simultaneous analysis of phenolic acids with mass spectrometric assay [9], and performance in eliminating uremic toxins such as albumin binding toxins [10], middle molecular substances, and small molecular proteins. The mechanism of dialysis-induced hypotension has been elucidated [11], and a method of blood volume monitoring has been developed [12]. Cell-wash dialysis [13], push-pull HDF [14], buttonhole cannulation and other methods have been developed as methods of removing substances with good efficiency. Such research and development has made it possible to eliminate target uremic toxins safely and efficiently. As mentioned below, it has become possible for people who choose HHD to choose from among many forms of treatment from the perspective of social life and treatment quality.

Diversification of Hemodialysis Therapy

Most hemodialysis therapy protocols in Japan use 3 sessions/week. One dialysis session is most commonly 4 h. However, Charra et al. [15] reported obtaining higher long-term survival rates with dialysis for 8 h/session 3 times/week. In Japan as well, dialysis of ≥6 h/session is recommended as long dialysis when dialysis is done 3 times/week. Pierratos et al. [16] perform nocturnal hemodialysis in which dialysis is done for 6–12 h at one time overnight, with an average of 8 h. Buttonhole cannulation is also widely used. In some protocols, dialysis is done ≥4 times/week.

According to a statistical survey by the Japanese Society for Dialysis Therapy, the optimum range for factors affecting the 1-year survival rate are as shown in table 1 when dialysis is done 3 times/week [17]. When dialysis is done 3 times/ week, results showed that the 1 year death rate was statistically significantly lower when a single session was ≥5 h than when it was <5 h. In Japan, however, the number of patients who undergo dialysis for ≥6 h/session is small, and they were not surveyed. The number of patients who undergo frequent dialysis of >4 times/week is also small, and the relationship with the death rate in a large number of patients is unknown. Scribner and Oreopoulos [18] proposed hemodialysis products as a better index of dialysis adequacy than Kt/V for use with diversifying dialysis methods.

Future Outlook for Home Hemodialysis

The long-term survival rate is higher with HHD than with dialysis in a medical facility for 4 h/session, 3 times/week. In Japan, the number of home

Table 1. Risk factors that affect the 1-year survival rate and the optimal range for each (with dialysis 3 times/week)

Risk factors	Optimal range
Dialysis time per session	≥5 h
Kt/V	≥1.6
Body weight increase in the first dialysis session of a week	4–6% of dry weight
Predialysis hematocrit value in the first dialysis session of a week	≥35%
Predialysis albumin concentration in the first dialysis session of a week	≥4.0 g/dl
Protein catabolic rate in the first dialysis session of a week	≥0.9 ≤1.1* (g/kg body weight/day)
Percent creatinine generation rate (% CGR) in the first dialysis session of a week	mortality rate decreases as % CGR becomes larger
Predialysis β_2-microglobulin concentration in the first dialysis session of a week	≤20 mg/l*

* These results were obtained from a stepwise logistic regression analysis of 71,746 people registered in the patient registry of the Japanese Society for Dialysis Therapy who fulfilled all the necessary requirements for this analysis [17].

Table 2. Key items that need to be improved for HHD therapy to spread in Japan

1   Reduction of the self-pay portion of expenses needed for partial renovation of the home and electric, water, and sewer facilities necessary for HHD
2   Reduction of the self-pay burden of electric and water fees needed for HHD
3   Thorough collection and treatment of medical waste by local governments
4   Payment of an allowance to caregivers
5   Promotion of a network for real-time distance management of information during HHD

dialysis patients who have continued dialysis treatments for more than 40 years is increasing. Home dialysis also has many advantages over hemodialysis in a medical facility in terms of activities of daily living and quality of life in social life. However, for it to spread further, the problems of current HHD shown in table 2 will need to be resolved.

HHD therapy has the major advantage that the treatment modality, such as the time per dialysis session and the number of sessions per week, can be changed to match the living circumstances of the individual. To guarantee the quality of the treatment effect however, a patient registry to evaluate treatment outcomes with various modalities and a mechanism to guarantee the results of analytical evaluations of those data are needed. It would seem to be proper to give that task to the statistical survey committee of the Japanese Society for Dialysis Therapy or the Japanese Home Dialysis Research Group.

Analysis of indictors for the adequacy of dialysis is not a simple problem, but other than survival rate, important issues for investigation are factors that affect complications and factors that affect itchiness, restless leg syndrome, insomnia, decreased appetite, and weight loss, which tend to occur when dialysis is insufficient. Moreover, among patients who undergo treatment for 6–8 h/session, 6 times/week, many express a feeling of exhilaration at the 'overflowing energy' in their body. Such frequent, long-duration treatment may be the ultimate optimal therapy, but it is also thought to be necessary to investigate the state of the intracellular environment with this kind of treatment.

With HHD it is easy to increase the number of dialysis sessions per week, and this modality occupies an important place as a modality with which diversified hemodialysis therapy can be achieved. Overcoming factors that are impediments to HHD to make it easier to increase HHD patients is important issue. If the above-mentioned registry of these patients and its analysis is properly done, the relationship between the body's internal environment and death or debilitation can be clarified. These results could be used not only in improving treatment for dialysis patients. The possibility that could play a role in slowing the decline in elderly people in general is also a major, important issue.

References

1 Maeda K: Haemodialysis in the home. Jpn J Nephrol 1971;13:116–119.
2 Maeda K, Kawaguchi S, Kobayashi K: Haemodialysis in the home – a progress report. Jpn J Nephrol 1972;14:31–34.
3 Watanabe Y, Nakamoto M, Chiba E, Hirano H, Akiba T, Kinugasa E, Ogawa H, Nakai S, Asano Y: Suggestions for home hemodialysis (in Japanese). J Jpn Soc Dial Ther 1998;31: 959–965.
4 Kobayashi K, Shibata M, Kato K, Nakamura S, Kato S, Kurachi K, Maeda K, Imai T, Yasuda B, Ohta K, Kawaguchi S, Tsutsui S, Shimizu K, Yamazaki C, Manji T, Nomura T: Extra corporeal ultrafiltration method: ECUM. Jpn J Nephrol 1972;14:539–553.
5 Ohta K, Shimoji A, Saito A, Maeda K, Kobayashi K, Fujisaki Y: Bemberg hollow fiber capillary kidney. Trans Am Soc Artif Int Organs 1973;19:98–104.
6 Maeda K, Ohta, Saito A, Shimoji T, Amano I, Manji T, Kawaguchi S, Kobayashi K, Fujisaki Y, Eiga S: ASAHI hollow fiber kidney: a progress report. Trans Am Soc Artif Int Organs 1974;20A:344–352.
7 Manji T, Maeda K, Kawaguchi S, Kobayashi K, Ohta K, Saito A, Amano I, Shimoji T, Fujisaki Y: Short time dialysis with 2 m² hollow fiber kidney. Proc Eur Dial Transplant Assoc 1974;11:153–157.
8 Yamamoto Y, Manji T, Maeda K, Ohta K: Ion-exchange chromatographic separation and fluorometric detection of guanidine compounds in physiologic fluids. J Chromatogr 1979;162:327–340.
9 Niwa T, Ohki T, Maeda K, Saito A, Kobayashi K: Quantitation of phenols and phenolic acids in uremic serum using gas chromatography-mass spectrometry. Proc Am Soc Mass Spectrometry 1980;28:284–285.

10 Niwa T, Takeda N, Maeda K, Shibata M, Tatematsu A: Accumulation of furancarboxylic acids in uremic serum as inhibitions of drug binding. Clin Chim Acta 1988;173: 127–138.

11 Maeda K, Morita H, Shinzato T, Vazquez Vega B, Kobayakawa H, Ishihara T, Inagaki H, Igarashi I, Kitano T: Role of hypovolemia in dialysis-induced hypotension. Artif Organs 1988;12:116–121.

12 Maeda K, Shinzato T, Yoshida F, Tsuruta Y, Usuda M, Yamada K, Ishihara T, Inagaki F, Igarashi I, Kitano T: Newly developed circulating blood volume-monitoring system and its clinical application for measuring changes in blood volume during hemofiltration. Artif Organs 1986;10:452–459.

13 Maeda K, Kawaguchi S, Kobayashi S, Niwa T, Kobayashi K, Saito A, Iyoda S, Ohta K: Cell-wash dialysis. Trans Am Soc Artif Int Organs 1980;26:213–218.

14 Usuda M, Shinzato T, Sezaki R, Kawanishi A, Maeda K, Kawaguchi S, Shibata M, Toyoda T, Asakura Y, Ohbayashi S: New simultaneous HF and HD with no infusion fluid. Trans Am Soc Artif Intern Organs 1982;28:24–27.

15 Charra B, Calemard E, Ruffet M, Chazot C, Terrat JC, Vanel T, Laurent G: Survival as an index of adequacy of dialysis. Kidney Int 1992;41:1286–1291.

16 Pierratos A, Ouwendyk M, Francoeur R, Vas S, Raj DS, Ecclestone AM, Langos M, Uldall R: Nocturnal hemodialysis. Three-year experience. J Am Soc Nephrol 1998;9:859–868.

17 Shinzato T, Nakai S, Akiba T, Yamazaki C, Sasaki R, Kitaoka T, Kubo K, Shinoda T, Kurokawa K, Marumo F, Sato T, Maeda K: Survival in long-term haemodialysis patients: results from the annual survey of the Japanese Society for Dialysis Therapy. Nephrol Dial Transplant 1996;11:2139–2142.

18 Scribner BH, Oreopoulos DG: The hemodialysis product: a better index of dialysis adequacy than Kt/V. Dial Transplant 2002;31: 13–15.

Kenji Maeda
Daiko-Sunadabashi Clinic, Fujita Health University School of Health Sciences
16-23 Daiko 4-chome,Higashi-ku
Nagoya-City, Aichi 461–0043 (Japan)
Tel. +81 52 711 8889, E-Mail ds.kenji.m@gmail.com

Suzuki H (ed): Home Dialysis in Japan.
Contrib Nephrol. Basel, Karger, 2012, vol 177, pp 106–116

Current International Status of Home Hemodialysis

Akira Saito[a,b] · Yoriko Ohta[a] · Kazuhiro Sato[a] · Mayuri Ichinose[a] ·
Tatsuro Arii[a] · Katsuhide Toyama[a]

[a]Yokohama Dai-ichi Hospital of Zenjin Foundation, Yokohama, and [b]Tokai University School of
Medicine, Isehara, Japan

Abstract

Three times weekly home hemodialysis (HHD) was introduced shortly after the initiation of chronic hemodialysis (HD) treatment in 1960. HHD eliminates the need of transportation to and from the dialysis unit and by allowing patients to set their own dialysis schedule, decreases the burden of treatment on their personal and professional lives. HHD has been found more economical and more highly associated with better patient survival than in-center dialysis. Nevertheless, the global prevalence of HHD decreased between 1980 and 2000 due to the increased availability of dialysis units and continuous ambulatory peritoneal dialysis, advances in cadaveric kidney transplantation, and several other factors. However, the availability of HHD at a frequency of more than 3 times/week, the typical frequency of conventional HD (CHD), in such forms as brief HD sessions of 2–3 h 5–6 days/week and nocturnal HD (NHD) has led to reversals in this trend. Frequent HHD, such as short daily HD (SDHD) and NHD instead of 3 times/week CHD, has been found to significantly improve hypertension, left ventricular mass, renal anemia, quality of life and mortality. On the other hand, NHD has been found to significantly improve hypertension, left ventricular mass, renal anemia, quality of life, malnutrition, mortality and phosphate clearance. Many observational clinical studies and one randomized controlled trial of SDHD and/or NHD have been conducted, and compact and convenient dialysis machines have been developed and used for HHD. The most recent data reported in the national and local registries of selected countries indicate that the prevalence of HHD among all dialysis patients from 2008 to 2010 varied from 0 to 3.3% except in New Zealand and Australia, where it was 16.3 and 9.3%, respectively. As HHD appears to be a more effective and economical dialysis modality than in-center CHD, its prevalence is likely to increase in the future.

Home hemodialysis (HHD) was initially introduced to overcome the difficulty experienced by renal failure patients in transportation to and from dialysis units, which had been thinly distributed among communities during the first stage of chronic hemodialysis (HD) treatment in the 1960s and 1970s. HHD also provides other advantages, including the self-scheduling of treatment, maintenance of privacy, provision of more time with family members, and reduced risk of infection from a dialysis unit. However, it also poses the disadvantages of requiring the services of a helper for self-dialysis, posing the risk of self-cannulation, requiring training in HD procedures, and requiring space to store dialysate, dialyzers, and other dialysis-related equipment and materials in the home. The prevalence of conventional hemodialysis (CHD) in the home has gradually decreased on a global scale with changes in circumstances surrounding HD therapy since 1980.

Nevertheless, the prevalence of HHD is increasing in the USA and several other countries, possibly because forms of HD that require frequent treatment, such as short daily home hemodialysis (SDHD) and nocturnal home hemodialysis (NHD), have been reported to be more effective and less symptomatic than CHD. This article describes the history, present status, advantages and disadvantages, and modalities of HHD currently used throughout the world.

History of Home Hemodialysis

HHD was first conducted by Nosé [1] in the USA in 1961. Scribner [2] trained a physician to look after the first patients to be treated by maintenance HD at home in 1963, 3 years after Quinton and Scribner [3] had developed an external shunt as a means of permanent vascular access, which made repeated HD treatments available for every chronic renal failure patient. HHD programs were subsequently developed by Merrill in Boston, Scribner in Seattle, and Shaldon in London between 1963 and 1964. HHD is currently available in developed countries, and has a high prevalence in Australia, New Zealand, Canada and some European countries. After reaching a high of 40% in the 1970s in the USA [4], the prevalence of HHD fell to 6% in the mid-1980s, and further fell to 0.62% in the 1990s [5]. The increasing age and comorbidity of dialysis patients, and an increase in several factors, including number of dialysis facilities, access to continuous ambulatory peritoneal dialysis, success in cadaveric kidney transplantation, and use of live donor kidney transplantation, have been suggested as the cause of the decline [6]. Above all, governmental cutbacks in funding for dialysis therapy might be the most important reason in encouraging a transition to HHD worldwide, as the number of dialysis patients has been growing worldwide.

In the 1980s, Buoncristiani et al. [7] treated patients with 2-hour sessions of SDHD treatment 6 times/week who failed to respond to CHD treatment. An

NHD program funded by the Ministry of Health of Ontario, Canada, was initiated in the 1990s. The clinical results of the studies reported by Uldall et al. [8] and subsequent studies affected the practices of dialysis physicians. As the clinical effectiveness of SDHD and NHD has become known to dialysis physicians worldwide, the number of SDHD and NHD patients has been gradually increasing. However, the prevalence of HHD in most countries remains very low, currently less than 3.3% of all dialysis patients, except Australia and New Zealand where its prevalence was 9.3 and 16.3%, respectively, in 2010 [9]. HHD has not been selected by many HD patients, nor has it been approved by the governments as a dialysis modality. In the USA, the prevalence of HHD slowly increased from 0.62% in 2005 to 1.0% in 2008. Based on their analysis of a 2010 questionnaire and the USRDS 2010 Report with a 3.1% growth rate, Blagg and Lockridge estimated the current prevalence of HHD in the USA at 1.6% (about 6,800 patients) [C.R. Blagg, pers. commun.]. According to the 2009 ERA-EDTA Registry, the prevalence of HHD in Europe was between 0 and 2.7% of all dialysis patients in 32 countries in 2009 [10].

In Japan, HHD has been used since it was first introduced in 1967 in Nagaya. At the first stage of HHD in Japan, end-stage renal failure patients who wanted to be treated with HD had to buy a batch-type dialysis machine, the Kiil-type dialyzer, and dialysis-related equipment with no financial assistance because the Japanese healthcare system did not cover dialysis treatment at that time. Although reimbursement for HHD by the healthcare system was approved by the Japanese Government in 1998, the prevalence of HHD remains very low at only 0.05% of all dialysis patients in 2007. The two main causes of the low prevalence may be that CHD patients have a good prognosis and high quality of life in Japan, compared to patients in other countries, and that dialysis units are available within 20–30 min at any location anywhere in Japan. HHD has recently gained attention among HD patients after the introduction of more frequent and/or longer HD treatments, as reflected by a slight increase in the prevalence of HHD patients to 0.1% in 2010 [11]. The prevalence of HHD from 2008 to 2010 in selected countries is shown in table 1.

Advantages of Conventional Home Hemodialysis

HHD is conducted as a form of 3 times/week CHD using the standard dialysis machines used in dialysis units. It has been shown that compared to in-center HD, CHD at home is cheaper [12, 13] and is associated with both better patient survival [14–17] and greater patient rehabilitation [16]. However, no randomized control trials (RCTs) comparing in-center and HHD patients have been conducted, and home CHD has been evaluated only in observational cohort studies.

Table 1. Prevalence of HHD among all dialysis patients in selected countries, 2008–2010

Country	HHD, %	Registry	Country	HHD, %	Registry
USA	1.0	USRDS 2010[1]	Italy	2.7	ERA-EDTA 2009
Argentina	0.0	USRDS 2010	Japan	0.1	JSDT Registry 2010[2]
Australia	9.3	ANZDATA 2010[3]	Malaysia	1.0	USRDS 2010
Austria	0	ERA-EDTA 2009[4]	Mexico	0	USRDS 2010
Bangladesh	0.3	USRDS 2010	New Zealand	16.3	ANZDATA 2010
Belgium	0.7	ERA-EDTA 2009	Philippines	0	USRDS 2010
Canada	3.5	CORR 2011[5]	Poland	0	ERA-EDTA 2009
Denmark	2.7	ERA-EDTA 2009	Spain	0.1	ERA-EDTA 2009
Finland	1.6	ERA-EDTA 2009	Serbia	1.3	USRDS 2010
Norway	0.1	ERA-EDTA 2009	Taiwan	0	USRDS 2010
Sweden	1.2	ERA-EDTA 2009	Thailand	0	USRDS 2010
Netherlands	1.0	ERA-EDTA 2009	UK	1.2	ERA-EDTA 2009
Hong Kong	0.41	USRDS 2010	Uruguay	0	USRDS 2010

[1] 2008 data as reported from the United States Renal Data System (USRDS) 2010.
[2] Japanese Society for Dialysis Therapy, present status of chronic dialysis in Japan on December 31, 2010.
[3] Australia and New Zealand Dialysis and Transplant 2010 Registry.
[4] European Renal Association-European Dialysis and Transplantation Association Annual Report 2009 Registry.
[5] Canadian Renal Replacement (CORR) 2011 Registry.

Advantages of More Frequent HHD

Moreover, almost all the clinical trials that described the benefits of SDHD and NHD were observational cohort studies, with few being RCTs or ongoing studies. The advantages reported in these studies are likely clinical advantages. To fill this research gap, RCTs should be conducted to compare SDHD and/or NHD with CHD in order to compare home CHD with in-center CHD. Lockridge [18] conducted the study of an NHD program with the largest number of participants, while Culleton et al. [19] performed the only randomized NHD study to have been reported to date in 2007. In the USA, SDHD and NHD programs with large numbers of participants were established by the Frequent Hemodialysis Network, with government funding in the 2000s.

Solute Clearances

In a randomized home nocturnal trial comparing 6 and 3 times/week CHD, the FNH found substantially greater differences between NHD patients and controls compared to daytime 6 times/week NHD patients and controls

Table 2. Advantages of HHD in comparison with conventional in-center HD

Conventional HHD		Short daily HHD		Nocturnal HHD	
Clinical advantages	ref.	clinical advantages	ref.	clinical advantages	ref.
Survival	13–17	blood pressure control	15, 23	blood pressure control	19, 24, 26
Rehabilitation	16	left ventricular hypertrophy	15, 23	left ventricular hypertrophy	19, 26
Cost-effectiveness	12, 13, 42	renal anemia	28	renal anemia	24, 26, 29
		survival	17, 30, 31, 34	survival	17, 32–34
		quality of life	16, 23	quality of life	19, 26, 30
		malnutrition	31	malnutrition	32
		mineral metabolism	36	mineral metabolism	19, 26, 37
		solute clearances	20, 22	solute clearances	20, 21
		sleep disorder	39	sleep disorder	38

regarding a wide range of parameters, such as ultrafiltration rate, $stdKt/V_{urea}$, generation rate $(Gn)_{urea}$ to time-averaged concentrations $(TACs)_{urea}$, normalized β_2-microblobulin $(\beta_2 M)$ Gn to TACs of $\beta_2 M$ [20]. Raj et al. [21] found that NHD increases $\beta_2 M$ removal as a result of the higher frequency and dialysis duration of HD. Goldfarb-Rumyantzev et al. [22] demonstrated that solute removal, including that of small and middle molecules larger than urea, was greater in SDHD and long-duration dialysis than in CHD.

Impact of Home Hemodialysis Therapies on Comorbid Conditions and Patient Variables

The clinical advantages of SDHD and NHD are summarized below, and clinical advantages of home CHD, SDHD and NHD are listed in table 2.

Blood Pressure
Multiple observational studies and one RCT trial showed improved blood pressure with fewer or no medications with both SDHD and NHD [19, 23, 24, 26]. One cross-sectional study demonstrated that frequent HD, SDHD and NHD are associated with less dialysis-induced myocardial stunning compared to CHD. This lower incidence of stunning may contribute to the improved outcomes associated with frequent HD therapies [25].

Left Ventricular Hypertrophy
One preliminary RCT using cardiac magnetic resonance imaging demonstrated that 6-times/week NHD improved left ventricular mass and reduced the need for blood pressure medication compared to 3 times/week CHD [19]. Several prospective studies that observed patients who had transitioned from CHD to SDHD or NHD using two-dimensional echocardiography found that these patients experienced reductions in left ventricular mass index [23, 26].

Renal Anemia
Several studies observed an increase in hematocrit and decrease in recombinant human erythropoietin (rHuEPO) requirement with an increase in hemoglobin concentration after conversion from CHD to SDHD [27–29]. 63 patients who transitioned to NHD showed increases in hemoglobin concentration and concomitant decreases in rHuEPO requirement compared to 32 self-care CHD control patients [29]. Several other observational studies observed elevated hemoglobin concentration and decreased rHuEPO dose after transition from CHD to NHD. However, one RCT conducted by Culleton et al. [19] did not find a significant difference in hemoglobin level between the control and treatment groups. A greater number of RCTs using a large number of cases should be conducted.

Quality of Life
Several prospective observational studies using a variety of self-assessment questionnaires, such as the 36-Item Short Form Health Survey (SF-36), Sickness Impact Profile, and Beck Depression Inventory, showed improvement of quality of life measures in patients who had converted from CHD to NHD [26, 30]. In their RCT, Culleton et al. [19] observed clinically and statistically significant improvements in selected kidney-specific domains of quality of life in NHD patients (p = 0.01 for effects of kidney disease and p = 0.02 for burden of kidney disease), but no difference from controls in overall quality of life as assessed using the EuroQol-5D index.

Malnutrition
Many observational studies have reported improvement of parameters of nutritional status, such as increases in serum albumin level after transition from CHD to SDHD or NHD. Several studies have also reported improvement in appetite, and increase in weight gain with NHD or quotidian HD [31]. In a prospective evaluation of nutritional intake of 15 consecutive patients who converted from CHD to NHD, Ipema et al. [32] reported significantly increased protein intake, as measured by both dietary intake journal and normalized protein catabolic rate, and phosphate intake after transition from CHD to NHD, but no increase in serum phosphate levels.

In an analysis of 247 NHD patients of the CANadian Slow Long nightly ExtEnded dialysis Programs (CAN-SLEEP), Pauly et al. [33] found that NHD is associated with excellent adverse event-free survival. Johanson et al. [34] studied survival and hospitalization among NHD and SDHD patients in comparison to propensity score-matched controls undergoing 3 times/week CHD and found that NHD is associated with significant reductions in risk of mortality and mortality or major morbid event when compared to CHD, as well as a reduced but non-significant risk of death among patients using SDHD compared to controls. However, they did not find a significant difference between NHD and SDHD patients and matched control cohorts regarding all-cause and specific hospitalizations of death. The findings of several other cohort studies supporting significant improvement in survival with frequent/extended HHD were compared to in-center CHD in Australia, New Zealand [17] and England [41].

Kjellstrand et al. [35] studied the influence of t and Kt/V on survival in 262 SDHD patients and found no association between Kt/V and survival, but found that four factors, i.e. age, weekly dialysis hours, HHD, and secondary renal disease, were independently associated with survival. These findings indicate that undergoing more than 15 h of HD per week maximizes survival in SDHD patients.

Other Clinical Complications

Several observational studies reported that phosphate removal was significantly increased in SDHD and NHD compared with CHD, and that patients no longer require phosphate binders and restriction of dietary phosphate on NHD therapies [32, 36, 37]. Conversion from CHD to NHD or SDHD is associated with improvements in sleep disorders, including sleep apnea, restless leg syndrome [38, 39]. Conversion from CHD to NHD is also associated with improvements of psychomotor efficiency and increases in attention and working memory [40].

Economic Assessment of Home Hemodialysis

Numerous studies have reported that home CHD and frequent HHD are less costly than conventional in-center HD [12, 13, 41]. Recently, Komenda et al. [42] attempted to create a standardized model based on systematic review of the available literature from Australia, Canada, and the UK regarding the costs of and common approaches for assessing direct medical and non-medical costs to determine the economic viability of providing HHD. They found that the modeled costs for SDHHD and NHHD were higher than both in-center and home CHD in the UK, while they were lower than in-center HD and higher than home CHD in Australia and Canada. The higher costs of frequent HHD compared to home CHD are due to higher consumable usage with higher dialysis frequency. More research into the long-term economic viability of providing conventional and frequent HHD and conventional in-center HD is required to conduct a more comprehensive comparison.

Home Hemodialysis Equipment and Systems

Medical staff use standard dialysis machines (a dialysate supply system) for performing HHD at dialysis units. Although many researchers have tried to develop compact and convenient dialysis machines for HHD, few machines can be used in the home.

Aksys PHD
Aksys developed the Aksys PHD as a personal HD system that allows dialyzer and tubing reuse by hot water disinfection. Although available on the US market for SDHD of HHD patients from August 2002 to January 2007, the Aksys PHD is no longer commercially available [43].

NxStage System One®
NxStage (Lawrence, Mass., USA) designed the System One® to be an innovative, flexible device that delivers HD, hemofiltration, and/or ultrafiltration therapies to patients with renal failure or fluid overload [44]. Smaller than CHD machines, this system uses 4- to 6-liter preformed bags of ultrapure dialysate. NxStage offers online sale of dialysate when patients require an increase in dialytic clearances. Recently, this system has become widely accepted mainly in the USA as a portable HD machine for the treatment of SDHD patients, with 6,000 patients reported to have used NxStage System One® in November 2011. The unique characteristics of this system include a highly automated system design with a drop-in cartridge to facilitate training and simple operation.

Renal Solutions Allient Hemodialysis System
Allient (Warrendale, Pa., USA) designed the Renal Solution Allient Sorbent Hemodialysis System, a sorbent cartridge-based system, to serve as a dialysis machine for 3- to 8-hour sessions of HHD. In this system, water is mixed with small packets of dry chemicals that convert to dialysate, which is then continuously generated by the sorbent cartridge in the system [45]. The system requires an electrical source and 6 liters of portable water. The number of home users of this system, however, is remarkably lower than that of the NxStage System One®.

References

1 Nosé Y: Home hemodialysis: a crazy idea in 1963: a memoir. ASAIO J 2000;46:13–17.

2 Blagg CR: The history of home hemodialysis: a view from Seattle. Home Hemodial Int 1997;1:1–7.

3 Quinton W, Dillard D, Scribner BH: Cannulation of blood vessels for prolonged hemodialysis. Trans Am Soc Artif Intern Organs 1960;6:104–113.

4 Blagg CR: A brief history of home hemodialysis. Adv Ren Replace Ther 1996;3:99–105.

5 United States Renal Dialysis System (USRDS) 2008 Annual Data Report. Bethesda, National Institutes of Health, National Institute of Diabetes and Digestive and Kidney Diseases, 2008, p 98.

6 MacGregor MS, Agar JWM, Blagg CR: Home haemodialysis – international trends and variation. Nephrol Dial Transplant 2006;21: 1934–1945.

7 Buoncristiani U, Quintaliani G, Cozzari M, Giombini L, Ragaiolo M: Daily dialysis: long-term clinical metabolic results. Kidney Int 1998;24(suppl):S130–S140.

8 Uldall R, Ouwendyk M, Francoeur R, Wallace L, Sit W, Vas S, Pierratos A: Slow nocturnal home hemodialysis. Adv Ren Replace Ther 1996;3:133–136.

9 Australia and New Zealand Dialysis and Transplant Registry 2010.

10 European Renal Association-European Dialysis and Transplantation Association Annual Report 2009 (EDTA) Registry.

11 Japanese Society of Dialysis Therapy (JSDT): Current Status of Chronic Dialysis Patients in Japan, December 31, 2010. Tokyo, JSDT, 2011.

12 Mackenzie P, Mactier RA: Home hemodialysis in the 1990s. Nephrol Dial Transplant 1998;13:1944–1948.

13 Mowatt G, Vale L, Perez J, Wyness L, Fraser C, MacLeod A, Daly C, Stearns SC: Systematic review of the effectiveness and cost-effectiveness, and economic evaluation, of home vs. hospital or satellite unit haemodialysis for people with end-stage renal failure. Health Technol Asses 2003;7:1–174.

14 Woods JD, Port FK, Stannard D, Blagg CR, Held PJ: Comparison of mortality with home hemodialysis and center hemodialysis: a national study. Kidney Int 1996;49: 1464–1470.

15 Saner E, Nitsch D, Descoeudres C, Frey FJ, Uchlinger DE: Outcomes of home hemodialysis patients: a case-cohort study. Nephrol Dial Transplant 2005;20:604–610.

16 Oberley ET, Schatell DR: Home hemodialysis: survival, quality of life, and rehabilitation. Adv Ren Replace Ther 1996;3:147–153.

17 Marshall MR, Hawley CM, Kerr PG, Polkinghorne KR, Marshall RJ, Agar JW, McDonald SP: Home hemodialysis and mortality risk in Australian and New Zealand populations. Am J Kidney Dis 2011;58: 782–793.

18 Lockridge RS Jr: Daily dialysis and long-term outcomes – the Lynchburg Nephrology NHHD experience. Nephrol News Issues 1999;13:16–23.

19 Culleton BF, Walsh M, Klarenbach SW, Mortis G, Scott-Douglas N, Quinn RR, Tonelli M, Donnelly S, Friedrich MG, Kumar A, Mahallati H, Hemmelgarn BR, Manns BJ: Effect of frequent nocturnal hemodialysis vs. conventional hemodialysis on left ventricular mass and quality of life. A randomized control trial. JAMA 2007;298:1291–1299.

20 Greene T, Daugirdas JT, Depner TA, Gotch F, Kuhlman M, on behalf of the Frequent Hemodialysis Network Study Group: Solute clearances and fluid removal in the Frequent Hemodialysis Network trials. Am J Kidney Dis 2009;53:835–844.

21 Raj DS, Ouwendyk M, Francoeur R, Pierratos A: Beta-2-microglobulin kinetics in nocturnal hemodialysis. Nephrol Dial Transplant 2000;15:58–64.

22 Goldfarb-Rumyantzev AS, Cheung AK, Leypoldt JK: Computer simulation of small-solute and middle-molecule removal during short daily and long-thrice weekly hemodialysis. Am J Kidney Dis 2002;40:1211–1218.

23 Fagugli RM, Pasini P, Pasticci F, Ciao G, Cicconi B, Buoncristiani U: Effects of short daily hemodialysis and extended standard hemodialysis blood pressure and cardiac hypertrophy: a comparative study. J Nephrol 2006;19:77–83.

24 Pierratos A: Nocturnal home haemodialysis: an update on a 5-year experience. Nephrol Dial Transplant 1999;14:2835–2840.

25 Jefferies HJ, Virk B, Schiller B, Moran J, McIntyre CW: Frequent hemodialysis schedule are associated with reduced levels of dialysis-induced cardiac injury (myocardial stunning). Clin J Am Soc Nephrol 2011;6: 1326–1332.

26 Walsh M, Culleton B, Tonelli M, Manns B: A systemic review of the effect of nocturnal hemodialysis on blood pressure, left ventricular hypertrophy, anemia, mineral metabolism, and health-related quality of life. Kidney Int 2005;67:1500–1508.

27 Woods JD, Port FK, Orzol S, Buoncristiani U, Young E, Wolfe RA, Held PJ: Clinical and biochemical correlates of starting 'daily' hemodialysis. Kidney Int 1999;55:2467–2476.

28 Ting GO, Kjellstrand C, Freitas T, Carrie BJ, Zarghamee S: Long-term study of high-comorbidity ESRD patients converted to short daily hemodialysis. Am J Kidney Dis 2003;42:1020–1035.

29 Schwartz DI, Pierratos A, Richardson RM, Fenton SS, Chan CT: Impact of nocturnal home hemodialysis on anemia management in patients with end-stage renal disease. Clin Nephrol 2005;63:202–208.

30 Cardone KE, Manley HJ, Grabe DW, Meola S, Hoy CD, Bailie GR: Quantifying home medication regimen changes and quality of life in patients receiving nocturnal home hemodialysis. Hemodial Int 2011;15:234–242.

31 Spanner E, Suri R, Heidenheim AP, Lindsay RM: The impact of quotidian hemodialysis on nutrition. Am J Kidney Dis 2003;42: 30–35.

32 Ipema KJ, van der Schans CP, Vonk N, de Vries JM, Westerhuis R, Duym E, Franssen CF: A difference between day and night: protein intake improves after the transition from conventional to frequent nocturnal home hemodialysis. J Ren Nutr 2011 (E-pub ahead of print).

33 Pauly RP, Maximova K, Coppens J, Asad RA, Pierratos A, Komenda P, Copland M, Nesrallah GE, Levin A, Chery A, Chan CT, on behalf of the CAN-SLEEP Collaborative Group: Patient and technique survival among a Canadian multicenter nocturnal hemodialysis cohort. Clin J Am Soc Nephrol 2010;5:1815–1820.

34 Johansen KJ, Zhang R, Huang Y, Chen S-C, Blagg CR, Goldfarb-Rumyantzev AS, Hoy CD, Lockridge Jr RS, Miller BW, Eggers PW, Kutner NG: Survival and hospitalization among patients using nocturnal and short daily compared to conventional hemodialysis: a USRDS study. Kidney Int 2009;76: 984–990.

35 Kjellstrand C, Buoncristiani U, Ting G, Traeger J, Piccoli GB, Sibai-Galland R, Young BA, Blagg CR: Survival with short-daily hemodialysis: association of time, site, and dose of dialysis. Hemodial Int 2010;14: 464–470.

36 Yuen D, Richardson RM, Chan CT: Improvements in phosphate control with short daily in-center hemodialysis. Clin Nephrol 2005;64:364–370.

37 Mucsi I, Hercz G, Uldall R, Ouwendyk M, Francoeur R, Pierrtoa A: Control of serum phosphate without any phosphate binders in patients treated with nocturnal hemodialysis. Kidney Int 1998;53:1399–1404.

38 Hanly PJ, Pierratos A: Improvement of sleep apnea in patients with chronic renal failure who undergo nocturnal hemodialysis. N Engl J Med 2001;344:102–107.

39 Jaber BL, Schiller B, Burkart JM, Daoui R, Kraus MA, Lee Y, Miller BW, Teitelbaum I, Williams AW, Finkelstein FO, on behalf of the FREEDOM Study Group: Impact of short daily hemodialysis on restless legs symptoms and sleep disturbances. Clin J Am Soc Nephrol 2011;6:1049–1056.

40 Jassal SV, Devins GM, Chan CT, Bozanovic R, Rourke S: Improvements in cognition in patients converting from thrice weekly hemodialysis to nocturnal hemodialysis: its impact on costs and quality of life. Am J Kidney Dis 2001;37:777–789.

41 Nitsch D, Steenkamp R, Tomson CR, Roderick P, Ansell D, MacGregor MS: Outcomes in patients on home haemodialysis in England and Wales, 1997–2005: a comparative cohort analysis. Nephrol Dial Transplant 2011;26:1670–1677.

42 Komenda P, Gavaghan MB, Garfield SS, Poret AW, Sood MM: An economic assessment model for in-center, conventional home, and more frequent home hemodialysis. Kidney Int 2012;81:307–313.

43 Kjellstrand CM, Blagg CR, Bower J, Twardowski ZJ: The Aksys personal hemodialysis system. Semin Dial 2004;17:151–153.

44 Scott A: Portable home hemodialysis for kidney failure. Issues Emerg Health Technol 2007;108:1–4.

45 Shu F, Parks R, Maholtz J, Ash S, Antaki JF: Multimodal flow visualization and optimization of pneumatic blood pump for sorbent hemodialysis system. Artif Organs 2009;33: 334–345.

Akira Saito, MD, PhD
Yokohama Dai-ichi Hospital of Zenjin Foundation
2-5-15, Takashima, Nishi-ku
Yokohama, Kanagawa 220-0011 (Japan)
Tel. +81 45 453 6711, E-Mail akira.saito@grp.zenjinkai.or.jp

Saito · Ohta · Sato · Ichinose · Arii · Toyama

Suzuki H (ed): Home Dialysis in Japan.
Contrib Nephrol. Basel, Karger, 2012, vol 177, pp 117–126

Future Home Hemodialysis – Advantages of the NxStage System One

Susumu Takahashi

NPO International Kidney Evaluation Association Japan, Tokyo, Japan

Abstract

To improve the quality of life (QOL) of patients with renal failure who are on dialysis, we have been working to promote home hemodialysis (HHD), but it has not come into widespread use at present because of various problems, including limitations of the equipment, the large proportion of elderly patients, and difficulty performing self-care. With regard to problems with the equipment, dialysis equipment for home use has not yet been approved in Japan, so equipment designed for medical facilities has to be used for home dialysis. Such equipment is bulky and occupies living space, as well as involving the cost of home renovation and the need for a caregiver. The NxStage System One (NSO) artificial kidney has served advantages for HHD compared with conventional equipment, since it is compact, portable, and easy to operate (especially for preparation and cleaning), does not require a water supply, occupies less living space, and reduces the need for renovation of the home. Other advantages of the NSO include improvement of QOL by saving time travelling to hospitals and helping patients to participate in social activities. In addition, HHD with the NSO can improve sleep disorders, the restless legs syndrome, and depressive symptoms, resulting in a good outcome. Moreover, HHD with the NSO reduces the need for drugs, such as antihypertensive medications and erythropoietin, possibly leading to saving of healthcare costs.

At present, about 300,000 people in Japan [1] and over 2.6 million people worldwide are suffering from end-stage renal disease (ESRD) and are being treated by dialysis or transplantation, and their number is expected to double within the next 10 years. There also seem to be more patients with predialysis chronic kidney disease.

While renal transplantation can provide a permanent solution to ESRD, long-term hemodialysis (HD) is still the mainstay of treatment. In Japan, about 10,000 recipients of kidney transplants still have functioning kidneys at present, and only about 20% of patients with ESRD have undergone kidney transplantation around the world [2]. Thus, most patients with ESRD undergo in-center HD (ICHD) 3 times weekly at an average annual cost of over JPY 5 million per patient, so dialysis treatment consumes a considerable proportion of healthcare resources.

Home hemodialysis (HHD) has been one of the options for treatment of ESRD for about 50 years, but the large size of the equipment, difficulties with its use, and other factors have prevented this treatment modality from gaining much popularity. The safety of home-based daily HD using the portable artificial kidney system NxStage System One (NSO, NxStage Medical Inc., Lawrence, Mass., USA) has been demonstrated in many countries around the world, and the clinical efficacy of short daily HHD with this new system has been recognized [3, 4]. The present report compares the profile of NSO with that of existing treatment modalities, and also introduces its features and the results of recent studies.

Current Treatment Modalities and Their Problems

Patients with acute or chronic renal failure depend on blood purification therapy to treat this life-threatening condition. At present, ICHD is the mainstay of treatment and patients undergo ICHD for about 3 times weekly with 4 h treatment on average. This means that dialysis patients have restrictions on their time and lifestyle, which interfere with social activities and reduce the quality of life (QOL). The travel time to and from hospital should also not be ignored. Furthermore, providing individual patients with an optimal (tailor-made) dialysis protocol is often difficult.

HHD has not become popular because of the problems with the size of conventional artificial kidney systems, difficulty with operation, and other factors. Continuous ambulatory peritoneal dialysis (CAPD) is another home therapy, but it has not become so popular because it cannot be continued over the long term due to deterioration of peritoneal function and because the equipment is difficult to operate. Accordingly, most patients are dependent on ICHD at present.

In Japan, current hospital dialysis equipment has been examined for efficacy and safety, but no HHD equipment has been approved by the Ministry of Health, Labor and Welfare. Accordingly, patients receiving HHD use the equipment designed for medical facilities in combination with a reverse osmosis system. Because the equipment is large, considerable living space is needed, which interferes with daily life. Also, many of the devices are noisy when operating, even though many patients perform HHD in their bedrooms or other rooms of their homes, and a large amount of waste is generated.

To promote HHD, a simple, compact, and portable device is needed in order to improve the QOL of patients, as well as the efficacy, safety, cost-effectiveness,

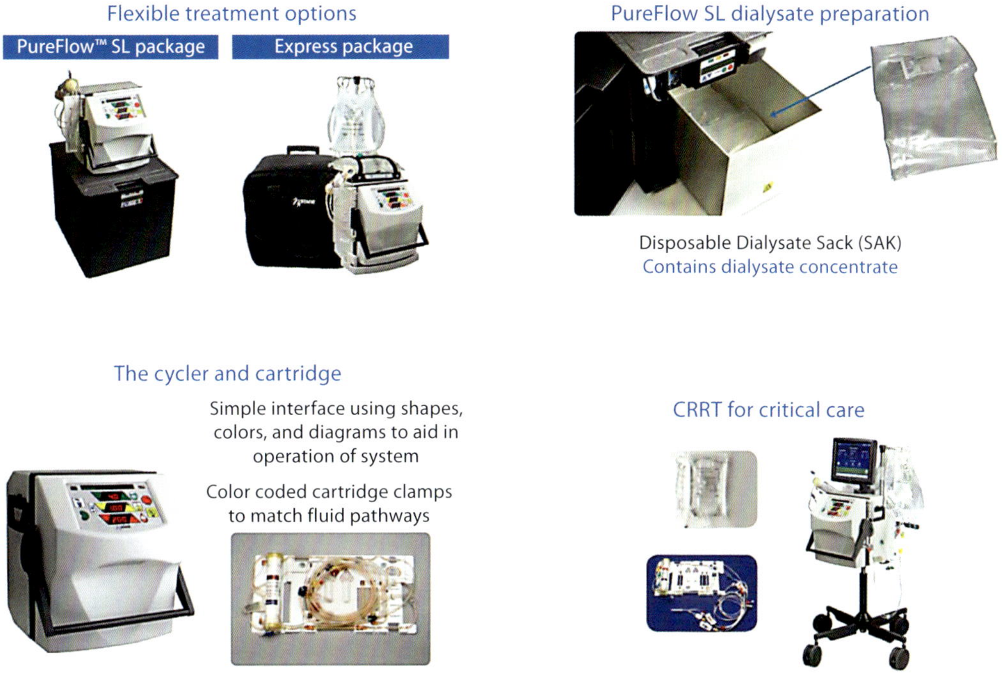

Fig. 1. System components for home treatment and acute care.

and environmental impact. Setting up a home for dialysis involves the cost of plumbing and other works, and disposal of wastes is always a problem. Since no kits have been approved for HHD, patients have been using those designed for medical facilities. However, preparation for dialysis and cleaning up after treatment are complicated procedures that take a long time.

NxStage Artificial Kidney System

The NxStage artificial kidney system comprises the NSO, PureFlow SL, NxStage Cartridge, and bagged dialysate. Figure 1 shows the components of the system for home treatment and for acute care. The device that controls the dialysis process is referred to as a cycler. It monitors treatment parameters and operating parameters that are important for safety, and also conducts pressure and alarm tests. The NSO can achieve a maximum blood flow rate of 600 ml/min and a maximum fluid exchange volume (dialysate volume + ultrafiltration volume) of 12 liters/h. The cycler removes blood from the patient and then returns the blood through a filter to the patient. The cycler is a portable device weighing about 30.5 kg and measuring 38.1 × 38.1 × 45.72 cm. It balances waste dialysate volume including ultrafiltration with the volume of incoming sterile dialysate (filled in a portable package). The cycler is equipped with a heater for warming dialysate.

The disposable gamma-sterilized NxStage Cartridge, with a preattached high-permeability filter, and a blood tube set. The cartridge, either with or without a filter, is easy to operate and is loaded into the cycler by a single step. Dialysate is usually supplied in a bag or prepared using NSO PureFlow SL™. When bagged dialysate is used, the dialysate is warmed with the NxStage Fluid Warmer, a component of the NSO that makes dialysis more comfortable. When dialysis is performed at a location where tap water is not available, bagged dialysate is generally used.

With regard to the dialysate composition, bicarbonate-based dialysate has mainly been used in Japan, and there is little experience with lactate-based dialysate. In contrast, lactate-based dialysate has been approved by the US FDA and its clinical safety has been reported [5].

The NSO is the control center of the system, since it regulates the blood flow through the dialyzer and the blood circuit and dialysate flow. The NSO is equipped with a special interface that allows an operator to control the flow rate according to the physician's instructions, monitors the system and ensures safety during treatment.

The NSO is an easy-to-operate, portable device that is equipped with dialysis monitoring and ultrafiltration functions. Since no liquids, including blood or dialysate, pass through the device, there is no need for disinfection of it and maintenance becomes easy. In addition, the NSO withstands tremor. Thus, the burden of performing HHD is reduced for patients because preparation and cleaning are simplified and less time is required. The schedule for performing HHD with the NSO is presented in figure 2 in comparison with that for a conventional device (the upper panel shows the schedule for the conventional device, and the lower panel is the schedule for the NSO). The NSO has solved the problem of a long time being required for preparation and for cleaning up after dialysis, thus approaching the ideal method of HHD and providing benefits for patients.

These advantages can also assist with the response to an emergency or disaster, since dialysis can be done anywhere if power is available. The NSO has the advantage of providing patients on HHD with more freedom, enabling them to travel for business or leisure by car or airplane. Figure 3 shows a car loaded with a complete NSO system.

Multiple Clinical Uses

In 2008, the United States Renal Data System (USRDS) reported that there were 3,826 patients on HHD in the USA [2] In February 2011, NxStage Medical Inc. announced that the NSO was being used by more than 5,000 patients around

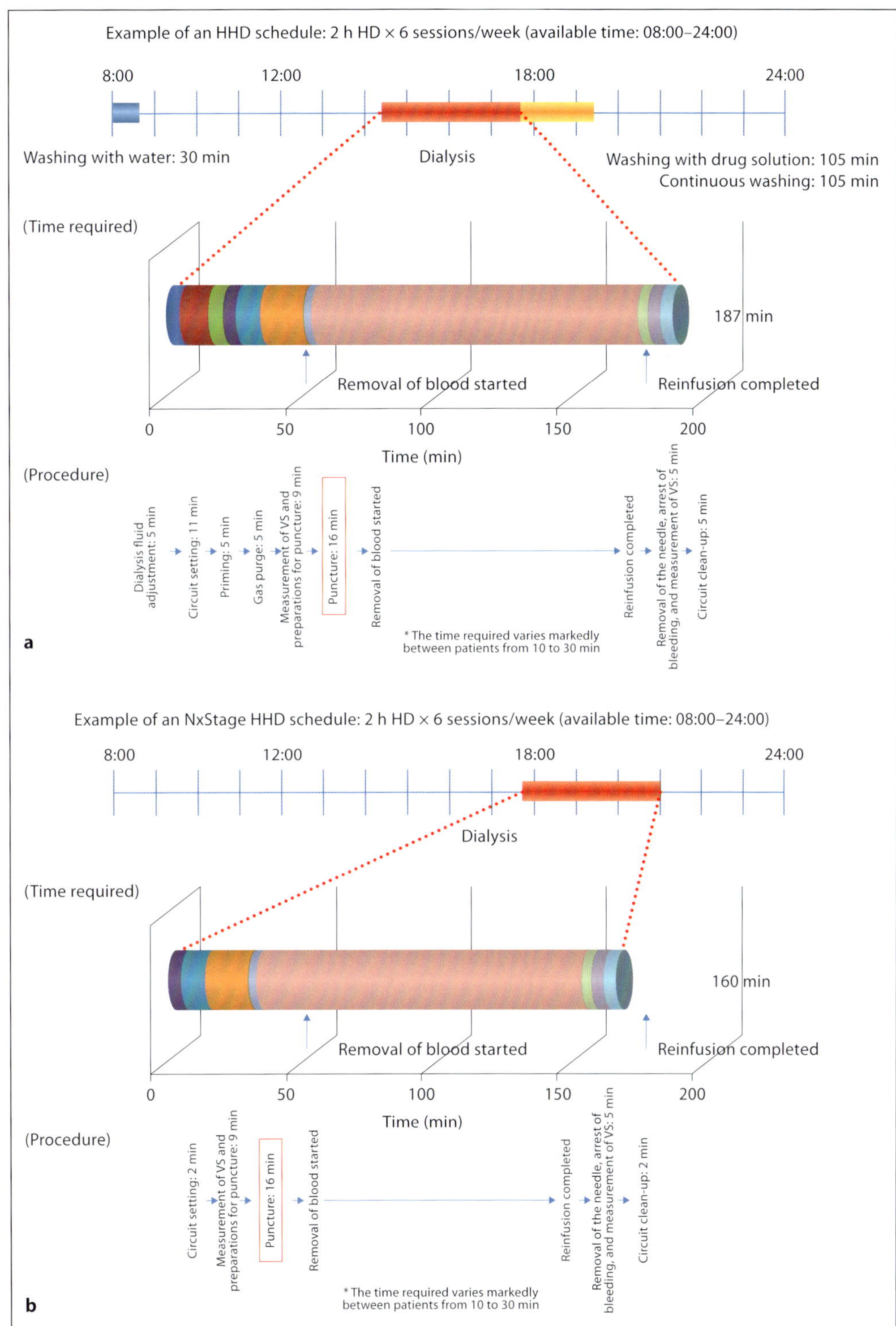

Fig. 2. Schedule for performing HHD with NSO.

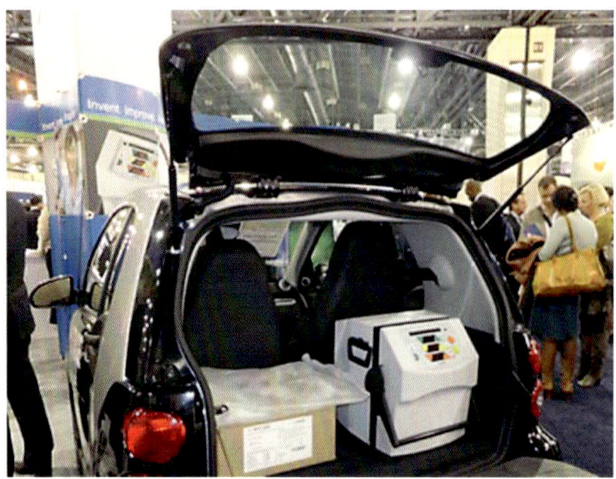

Fig. 3. Complete NSO system loaded in the back of a car.

the world, mainly in the USA, and that more than 4 million dialysis sessions had been performed.

According to a survey performed by the Japanese Society for Dialysis Therapy, only 279 patients were on HHD in Japan at the end of 2010, but this was an 18% increase compared with the number at the end of 2009 (229 patients). CAPD is another modality for home dialysis, and it was being used by 9,728 patients, among whom 628 had continued it for 5 years from 2005 [1]. It is assumed that some patients would wish to change to HHD after 5 years of CAPD and loss of their peritoneal function, but they may have to switch to ICHD because of the bulky equipment and complicated procedures. Since a small, easy-to-operate HD unit is not available in Japan at present, many patients on CAPD whose peritoneal function deteriorates have no choice but switch to ICHD, even if they wish to continue home dialysis.

With regard to continuing dialysis therapy in times of disaster, the impact was minimized after the Mid-Niigata Earthquake and the Great East Japan Earthquake by prompt patient transport and other countermeasures. There were few reports of fatalities among patients on HHD. Due to the advantages of being portable and not requiring running water or disinfection after the procedure, the NSO could be very effective for use both inside and outside the disaster zone, and could be loaded onto rescue craft in the future.

The NSO may also be used in intensive care units or for critical cases. It can be easily employed for the treatment of rhabdomyolysis and other similar conditions or for acute renal failure and such problems. The NSO has a volume control system that is not affected by movement, temperature, or the fluid volume, unlike a conventional scale-based continuous renal replacement therapy (CRRT) system. When the flow of fluid is restricted in any way, a closed system

Takahashi

Table 1. Currently available NSO cyclers and NSO PureFlow SL

	NSO cycler for home use	NSO cycler chronic/acute model for clinical setting	NSO PureFlow SL
USA (FDA approvals)			
USA	○	○	○
Europe CE mark approval			
	NSO cycler for home use	NSO cycler chronic/acute model for clinical setting	NSO PureFlow SL
Denmark	○		○
Finland	○		○
Italy	○		○
Netherlands	○	○	○
UK	○	○	○
Sweden	○		○
Other countries			
	NSO cycler for home use	NSO cycler chronic/acute model for clinical setting	NSO PureFlow SL
Canada	○	○	○
Australia	○	○	○
New Zealand	○	○	○
Saudi Arabia	○		

automatically sounds an alarm and stops to minimize imbalances. The NSO allows simplified management of fluids and can achieve the fluid removal prescribed for CRRT without the need for scales or a waste reservoir bag, which saves resources (fig. 1).

The NSO and PureFlow SL have already been used clinically in many countries, including the USA, Europe, Canada, and Australia (table 1). Early introduction of the NxStage system in Japan will be useful for the treatment of renal failure. We expect that this system will improve both the survival and QOL of patients with renal failure.

Indications for HHD

Since HHD is performed by the patient or caregiver without any healthcare professionals, an adequate support system is necessary. For performance of HHD, an appropriate system must be established according to the criteria for claiming treatment-specific medical fees. Only those patients who meet the following

personnel are not always present, ensuring safety so that accidents do not occur is of utmost importance. For this purpose, establishment of a training system to start HHD, an emergency handling and support system, and a system for maintenance checks of the reverse osmosis system and personal dialysis machine is essential.

Advantages and Disadvantages of HHD (Compared with Center Hemodialysis)
Advantages of HHD include that (1) dialysis can be tailored to suit family life, (2) the dialysis schedule can be freely made, (3) there are almost no time limitations when reintegrating into society, and (4) much time can be spent with the family during dialysis.

Disadvantages of HHD include that (1) a fixed period of time for training is needed together with the caregiver, (2) response is delayed during emergencies, (3) family understanding and cooperation are essential, and a caregiver is needed, and (4) construction expenses at the start of HHD and subsequent maintenance and operation costs (water, electricity, delivery) are incurred.

HHD Patient Number, and Their Proportion among Chronic Dialysis Patients
According to an overview of regular dialysis treatment in Japan by the dialysis survey committee of the Japanese Society for Dialysis Therapy, the number and proportion of HHD patients is increasing each year. As of the end of December 2010, the number was reported to be 279 (0.094%), although that was still less than 0.1% [1]. Factors in its slow spread in Japan may include that it is not well known by patients and health professionals, and that patients require a caregiver.

HHD Patients at Shinseikai Dai-ichi Hospital – Investigation of Dialysis
Situation and Daily Life, Circulatory Dynamics, and Nutritional Status
In an investigation of 36 HHD patients registered at out hospital in March 2008, there were 32 men (88.9%) and 4 women (11.1%), with a mean age of 51.3 ± 11.5 years. Mean dialysis history was 16.5 ± 12.3 years, with the longest being 39 years and 9 months. Nine patients (25.0%) had a dialysis history of ≥30 years, and 31 patients (86.1%) were employed and active in society. The caregiver was the patient's wife in 88.8% of cases, followed by husband in 5.6% and mother in 5.6%.

The dialysis schedule was every-other-day dialysis in 25 patients (69.4%) and 3 times/week in 11 patients (30.6%). Mean dialysis time was 5.1 ± 2.7 h/session and 17.0 ± 2.7 h/week, which is calculated to be about 1 session/week longer than standard dialysis administered in medical facilities.

Rate of body weight gain was 3.2 ± 1.2% and mean blood pressure was 98.1 ± 14.7 mm Hg before dialysis and 87.8 ± 17.0 mm Hg after dialysis. Thus, there was almost no blood pressure variation and HHD may be viewed as complaint-free dialysis.

In cardiovascular function, left ventricular ejection fraction was good at 68.0 ± 9.4%, and cardiothoracic ratio was 46.0 ± 4.9%. Albumin was 3.8 ± 0.4 g/dl and creatinine (Cr) index was 97.0 ± 18.0, showing good nutritional status. Dialysis dose (Kt/V) was 1.50 ± 0.25. With respect to anemia, hematocrit was 32.0 ± 3.8%, and 21 patients (58.3%) received an erythropoietin or darbepoietin treatment.

The Direction We Want to Pursue

Hemodialysis Product (HDP)
HDP was 57.3 ± 12.0 in 36 HHD patients in our hospital in March 2008. This value is higher than the borderline value (HDP 45) seen in the HDP table of Scribner and Scribner [2] but lower than the adequate value (HDP 72). With every-other-day HD for 5 h/session, HDP was 61.25, but with every-other-day HD for 6 h/session HDP was 73.5, close to the HDP 72 of Charra et al. [3]. How does vital prognosis change? The relationship between HDP and vital prognosis will probably be investigated in the future, but this will likely require consideration of how we should approach HD frequency.

Choices for HHD – From Short-Duration (Frequent) HD to Long-Duration (Frequent) HD
In recent years both long- and short-duration frequent dialyses have been reported to be effective in lowering mortality rate and improving vital prognosis (table 1). Starting in about 1970, Charra et al. [3] conducted prolonged slow hemodialysis (PHD) for 8 h, 3 times/week in Tassin, France. In Canada, Pierratos et al. [4] perform nocturnal hemodialysis (NHD; nighttime, long-duration, frequent hemodialysis) for 8–10 h, 6–7 times/week. In Perugia, Italy, Buoncristiani et al. [5] perform daily short dialysis (DHD) for 1.5–2 h on 7 consecutive days/week. Also in Italy, Mastrangelo et al. [6] in Lecce started performing frequent dialysis for 3 h, 5 times/week (Lecce dialysis: LHD) in 1978.

These dialysis treatments have a rather good vital prognosis compared with standard dialysis of 4 h/day, 3 days/week, and may be considered treatment options in the coming years. Ideal dialysis needs to efficiently clear uremic toxins of small- to middle-molecular weight and larger molecules, and to keep the peak value down. With the use of these methods, a high albumin value can be maintained and good phosphate control, high Kt/V and low β_2-microglobulin can be achieved. Improvements in left ventricular hypertrophy, hypertension, and left cardiac function have also been reported. Turning to survival rates, with the PHD of Charra et al. [3], the 10-year survival rate was 75.0%, 15-year survival rate was 55.0%, and 20-year survival rate was 43.0%. With LHD of Mastrangelo et al. [6], the 10-year survival rate was 60.0% and the 15-year survival rate was 48.0%. Comparing these results with data from the patient survey committee of the Japanese Society for Dialysis Therapy [1], PHD and LHD are seen to be clearly better (table 2).

Table 1. Reports on long- and short-duration frequent dialyses

	PHD Charra et al. [3]	NHD Pierratos et al. [4]	DHD Buoncristiani et al. [5]	LHD Mastrangelo et al. [6]
Dialysis duration, times/session	8	8–10	1.5–2	3
Dialysis frequency, sessions/week	3	6–7	7	5
Type of dialyzer	Cuprophan	PS	PAN	AN69, PMMA, PS
Area of dialyzer, m²	1.1–2.2	0.7–1.8	1.0	1.4–2.0
Dialysate volume, ml/min	500	100–200	1,200–1,500	500–800
Blood flow, ml/min	200–220	250–300	275	>300
Dialysis dose, Kt/V	$(1.67 \pm 0.41) \times 3$/week	$(1.00 \pm 0.23) \times (6\text{–}7)$/week	2.4–3.6/week	4.8 ± 0.75/week
Serum albumin level concentration	4.16	4.1 ± 0.3	–	3.97 ± 0.6
DPI, g/kg/day	1.33 ± 0.42	1.4 ± 0.2	–	1.32 ± 0.3

DPI = Diet protein intake; PAN = polyacrylonitrile; PMMA = polymethylmethacrylate; PS = polysulfone.

Table 2. Survival rates with long- and short-duration frequent dialyses

	PHD Charra et al. [3]	LHD Mastrangelo et al. [6]	JSDT Dialysis Survey Committee (December 2011)
Dialysis duration (times/session)	8	3	–
Dialysis frequency (sessions/week)	3	5	–
10-Year survival rate	75.0	60.0	36.1
15-Year survival rate	55.0	48.0	23.1
20-Year survival rate	43.0	–	17.1

According to a report by Raj, Charra et al. [7], left cardiac hypertrophy was seen in 76% of patients who underwent dialysis for 8 h, 3 times/week for 10 years or more. As one problem, they raised the question of whether a dialysis schedule that requires more frequent dialysis is necessary. We have recommended at least every-other-day dialysis. Considering caregiver burden and the time required for dialysis preparation and completion with current dialysis equipment, every-other-day dialysis, for example every other day with HD time of 5–6 h, would seem reasonable.

From a comparison of the survival rate of patients who underwent daily HHD, patients who underwent daily center hemodialysis, and patients who underwent 3 times/week hemodialysis in medical facilities in USA, it was reported that the survival rate was better in the daily HHD patients than in the daily center hemodialysis or 3 times/week hemodialysis patient, and that the 10-year survival rate was about the same as for patients who underwent cadaveric renal transplantation [8].

Nutritional Assessment Based on Geriatric Nutritional Risk Index (GNRI)
GNRI has been proposed as an indicator of nutrition in healthy elderly people; on the other hand, Yamada et al. [9] assessed nutrition in HD patients using GNRI and reported that a good nutritional state of GNRI among them is ≥92. In healthy elderly people, GNRI for a good nutritional state is ≥99 [10]. Among the 36 HHD patients at our hospital in March 2008, mean GNRI in 34 (excluding 1 patient with liver cancer and 1 patient with kidney cancer) was 97.4 ± 5.5. GNRI was ≥92 in 28/34 patients (82.4%), however the percentage of patients with GNRI of ≥99 dropped to below 40% (13/34; 38.2%). Nutritional status is an important problem, and improvements should be made in the future.

Conclusion

The major advantage of HHD is the degree of freedom in dialysis. HHD is done in settings near to daily life, and is convenient in terms of eating habits, family life, and social life (activities). It also contributes to higher quality of life. This means that HHD can be done in a style suited to the individual HHD patient. Schedules from short-duration frequent dialysis to long-duration (frequent) dialysis are possible. The main characteristic of HHD may be its diversity. Finally, HHD is thought to lead to improvements in nutritional state, physical and mental state, and vital prognosis. This is the direction in which we would like to take HHD.

References

1 Dialysis Survey Committee of the Japanese Society for Dialysis Therapy: An overview of regular dialysis treatment in Japan as of December 31, 2010, 2011, 2–22.
2 Scribner BH, Orepoiulos DG: The hemodialysis product: a better index of dialysis adequacy than Kt/V. Dial Transplant 2001;31: 13–15.
3 Charra B, Calemaral E, Ruffet M, et al: Survival as an index of adequacy of dialysis. Kidney Int 1992;41:1286–1291.
4 Pierratos A, Ouwendyk M, Vas S, et al: Nocturnal hemodialysis three years' experience. J Am Soc Nephrol 1998;9: 859–868.

5 Buoncristiani U, Glombini I, Cozzari M, et al: Daily recycled bicarbonate dialysis with polyacrylonitrile. ASAIO J 1983;29:669–672.

6 Mastragelo F, Alfonso M, Napoli V, et al: Diary with increased frequency of session (Lecce dialysis). Nephrol Dial Transplant 1998;13(suppl 6):S139–S147.

7 Raj DSC, Charra B, Pierratos A, Work J, et al: In search of ideal hemodialysis: is prolonged frequent dialysis the answer? Am J Kidney Dis 1999;34:597–610.

8 Kjellstrand CM, Buonocristiani U, Ting G, et al: Short daily haemodialysis: survival on 415 patients treated for 1,006 patient-years. Nephrol Dial Transplant 2008;23:3283–3289.

9 Yamada K, Furuya R, Takita T, et al: Simplified nutritional screening tools for patients on maintenance hemodialysis. Am J Clin Nutr 2008;87:106–113.

10 Bouillanne O, Morineau G, Dupont C, et al: Geriatiric Nutritional Risk Index: a new index for evaluating at-risk elderly medical patients. Am J Clin Nutr 2005;82:777–783.

Hiroshi Ogawa
Shinseikai Dai-ichi Hospital, 1-3-2 Tamamizu-cho
Nagoya 477-8633 (Japan)
E-Mail hrsogw@shinseikai.org

Suzuki H (ed): Home Dialysis in Japan.
Contrib Nephrol. Basel, Karger, 2012, vol 177, pp 133–142

Overnight Home Hemodialysis: Eight Patients and Six Years of Experience in Sakairumi Clinics

Hiroshi Tanaka[a] · Rumi Sakai[a] · Tomoyuki Kita[b] ·
Kumi Okamoto[b] · Maki Mikami[b]

[a]Medical Foundation Sakairumi Clinic Ashiya Sakairumi Clinic, Ashiya, and [b]Medical Foundation Sakairumi Clinic Sakairumi Clinic, Nadaku, Kobe, Japan

Abstract

We started our home hemodialysis (HHD) program in July 2005 and have been promoting overnight HHD. As more than 6 years have passed since we started our HHD program, we review our HHD program and 8 overnight HHD patients (5 males and 3 females). Their underlying disease differs in each and none have diabetic nephropathy. Their average age was 49.2 ± 6.0 years (mean $\pm$ SD). Average duration of dialysis treatment, HHD, and overnight HHD was 9.4 ± 4.4, 3.5 ± 2.4, and 2.2 ± 1.7 years, respectively. Average treatment time per dialysis session was 6.9 ± 0.8 h/treatment, average treatment days weekly was 4.5 ± 0.8 days/week, and average treatment time weekly was 31.2 ± 7.0 h/week. Laboratory data were good and their blood pressure was well controlled without any antihypertensive drugs excluding a patient who was recently introduced to dialysis with some residual kidney function. Severe problems did not occur in these 6 years except for blood access infection twice, slipping out of a needle during dialysis with small blood loss once, and a drop in blood pressure at the end of dialysis once, which was recovered by her assistant's help. According to our HHD training program, the average training duration for HHD was 106 ± 42 days. The shortest was 60 days and longest 198 days. These differences among training durations might be because of the frequency of training and having a better hand of puncturing. We did not instruct any additional issues and points for overnight HHD, because performing overnight HHD is similar to standard HHD. Some patients moved to overnight HHD slowly starting with once weekly and the others started overnight HHD several days after they had started HHD.

After the hemodialysis system was developed for humans by Kolff and Berk [1] in 1943, home hemodialysis (HHD) was started in 1964 by Scribner et al. [2] in

Seattle, by Merill et al. [3] in Boston, and by Shaldon [4] in London. At that time, hemodialysis systems such as the dialyzer, dialysis machine, dialysis fluid were not well developed compared with recent systems. Furthermore, Shaldon et al. [5] started overnight HHD in London in the following year in 1965. Afterwards, the number of HHD patients increased in the USA and Europe. On the other hand, the Japanese government was not interested in home treatment including hemodialysis after hemodialysis treatment was introduced in Japan. HHD was registered by the Japanese government in April 1998. It was very late compared with other countries that Japanese dialysis patients started HHD legally. The number of HHD patients in Japan did not increase and the number of HHD patients in Japan was 279, which accounted for 0.1% of all dialysis patients at the end of 2009 [6]. Overnight HHD was not easily accepted in Japan because hospitals which had the HHD program did not allow their patients to do dialysis at midnight.

We started our HHD program in July 2005 and our first HHD patient started his first treatment on November 30, 2005. We have been promoting overnight HHD among our patients because it can save a lot of time. It has been 40 years since Shaldon started overnight HHD. The number of overnight HHD patients has been increasing and as of November 30, 2011 we now have 8 patients. As more than 6 years have passed since we started our HHD program, we review our HHD program and overnight HHD patients.

Patients

Table 1 shows the profile of our 8 overnight HHD patients. Their average age was 49.2 ± 6.0 years (mean ± SD), which is younger than all our dialysis patients (60.0 years) in Ashiya Sakairumi Clinic and all Japanese dialysis patients (65.8 years) [6]. They are younger and more active and have their daytime jobs including a housewife. Male patients make up most of our patient group. Their underlying disease differs in each: there are 3 chronic nephritis patients, 2 polycystic kidney patients, 2 IgA nephropathy patients, and 1 chronic glomerulonephritis patient. None of them is a diabetic nephropathy patient. Their average duration of dialysis treatment in total was 9.4 ± 4.4 years. The longest was 16.8 years and shortest 0.8 years. Three patients used to be on continuous ambulatory peritoneal dialysis (CAPD) for 2.2–4.8 years. Their average duration of HHD is 3.5 ± 2.4 years. The longest is 7.8 years and the shortest 0.5 year. Their average duration of overnight HHD was 2.2 ± 1.7 years. The longest was 5.2 years and the shortest 0.5 year. Average treatment time per dialysis session was 6.9 ± 0.8 h, average treatment days weekly was 4.5 ± 0.8 days, and average treatment time weekly was 31.2 ± 7.0 h. The starting time of overnight HHD depends on lifestyle. As is easily understood, the above data, treatment hours, frequency, and starting time of treatment were not fixed. They did it from one day to the next according to their daily lifestyle. Overnight dialysis started at 22:30–24:00 h.

Dialysis Method

Our overnight HHD patients used high-flux dialyzers, whose mean membrane dimensions were 2.0 ± 0.3 m^2 (1.5–2.2 m^2) and whose β_2-microglobulin (β_2-MG) clearance was >50 ml/min. Mean blood flow rate was 201 ± 55 ml/min (130–270 ml/min). Dialysis fluid flow was mainly 500 ml/min, some patients set 350–400 ml/min.

Laboratory Data

Table 2 shows recent laboratory data of our overnight HHD patients. As everybody understands clearly, their laboratory data were very good. Their mean hemoglobin level was 11.0 ± 1.0 g/dl. Potassium level was very low without any polystyrene sulfonate for all patients. Mean total protein was 6.7 ± 0.4 g/dl and mean serum albumin was 4.3 ± 0.3 g/dl, which were higher than those of standard hemodialysis patients. BUN was lower compared with that of standard dialysis patients but serum creatinine was not so low. Serum calcium level was well controlled by taking activated vitamin D_3 in most of the patients. Serum phosphate level was also well controlled with some patients having phosphate binders. On the other hand, the lowest serum phosphate level among them was 1.8 mg/dl. Although we could not see any clinical abnormalities in those patients whose serum phosphate levels were very low, we prescribed two tablets of VisiClear combination tablets (Zeria Pharmaceutical Co. Ltd, Tokyo, Japan) containing 734.7 mg monobasic sodium phosphate monohydrate and 265.3 mg dibasic sodium phosphate anhydrous before dialysis to case 7.

The mean serum β_2-MG level was 17.9 ± 3.6 mg/l, which was much lower compared with that of standard dialysis patients. When we looked at the dialyzers being used, only case 2 was using a super high-flux dialyzer, i.e. APS-15E (1.5 m^2, polysulfone; Asahi Medical, Tokyo, Japan) whose β_2-MG clearance was >70 ml/min. The other patients were also using a high-flux dialyzer whose β_2-MG clearance was between 50 and 70 ml/min. The serum β_2-MG of case 2 was 20.2 mg/l, which was the second highest among them. Serum intact PTH level was well controlled for all patients, although cinacalcet hydrochloride was prescribed for 3 patients. We have the data of blood gas analysis in 3 patients, who had overnight hemodialysis in our clinic, before and after dialysis. Their dialysis time was 6–8 h. Serum bicarbonate level was 23.3 ± 2.3 mEq/l before dialysis and 28.1 ± 1.2 mEq/l afterwards. Dialysis fluids were Kindary AF2 and AF3 (Fuso Pharmaceutical Industries, Ltd, Osaka, Japan) whose bicarbonate level was set at 27.5 mEq/l (between 25 and 30 mEq/l). They were the same as those used by our overnight HHD patients. These data tell us that overnight HHD patients might have a similar change in serum bicarbonate.

Table 1. Patient profile of our overnight HHD patients (case 2 underwent his HHD training in another clinic before coming to us)

Case	Sex	Age	Underlying disease	Target body weight, kg
1	M	49.7	IgA nephropathy	81.5
2	M	42.5	chronic nephritis	77.0
3	M	38.6	chronic glomerular nephritis	74.5
4	F	51.9	polycystic kidney	43.0
5	M	48.0	IgA nephropathy	63.2
6	F	56.3	polycystic kidney	50.5
7	F	57.3	chronic nephritis	53.0
8	M	49.0	chronic nephritis	72.0
	Mean	49.2		64.4
	SD	6.0		13.2

Table 2. Laboratory data of our overnight HHD patients before dialysis

Case	RBC	WBC	Hb	Ht	Platelets	Na	K
1	450	4,900	11.9	41.8	22.0	139	4.8
2	358	5,900	10.6	34.2	25.2	141	3.9
3	387	5,400	12.0	40.7	24.0	139	4.3
4	333	3,600	10.1	31.0	18.4	139	3.7
5	320	5,100	10.3	32.0	18.5	141	4.7
6	380	4,500	11.2	36.4	22.3	142	4.7
7	388	4,600	10.3	34.3	16.0	142	4.2
8	359	3,200	11.2	33.0	17.6	134	5.5
Mean	372	4,650	11.0	35.4	20.5	140	4.5
SD	40	896	0.7	4.0	3.3	3	0.6

TP = Total protein; Alb = albumin; Cr = creatinine; i-P = inorganic phosphate; β_2-MG = β_2-microglobulin; i-PTH = intact-parathyroid hormone unit; RBC = $\times 10^6$/mm^3; WBC = /mm^3; Hb = g/dl; Ht = %; platelet = $\times 10^3$/mm^3; Na; K; Cl = mEq/l; TP; Alb = g/dl; BUN; Cr; Ca; i-P = mg/dl; β_2-MG = mg/l; i-PTH = pg/ml.

Blood Pressure and Some Symptoms during Overnight HHD and Some Other Problems

As their removal water rate per hour was smaller than that of conventional 3 times weekly 4-hour dialysis, a drop in blood pressure did not occur. Our patients had

Duration of dialysis, years			Training days of HHD	Overnight HHD performed		
total including CAPD	HHD	overnight HHD		h/week	h/session	days/week
10.4	6.0	5.2	133	27.4	6.3	4.4
9.5	7.8	4.4	–	36.2	7.5	4.8
16.8	5.1	2.9	102	28.6	7.8	3.7
8.4	3.1	0.7	193	41.4	8.2	5.1
5.6	2.3	1.7	86	28.1	6.4	4.4
11.6	1.7	1.7	60	24.2	6.2	3.9
12.2	1.4	0.7	101	41.3	6.6	6.2
0.8	0.5	0.5	69	22.2	6.0	3.7
9.4	3.5	2.2	106	31.2	6.9	4.5
4.4	2.4	1.7	42	7.0	0.8	0.8

Cl	TP	Alb	BUN	Cr	Ca	i-P	β_2-MG	i-PTH
100	6.6	4.4	55	10.8	9.6	6.2	22.2	260
103	6.5	4.1	44	10.8	9.2	4.5	20.2	153
104	7.0	4.4	44	9.2	10.2	3.3	18.8	28
103	6.4	4.0	25	4.4	9.4	2.5	14.1	163
102	7.4	4.9	50	9.0	8.8	1.8	19.9	69
107	6.5	4.3	48	6.1	9.1	3.4	20.7	217
103	6.4	4.0	14	4.1	8.9	2.1	12.3	76
97	6.5	4.4	43	8.4	9.2	4.3	14.7	108
102	6.7	4.3	40	7.8	9.3	3.5	17.9	134
3	0.4	0.3	14	2.7	0.4	1.5	3.6	79

to check their body weight, appetite, blood pressure, and consulted us about their target body weight. Their blood pressure before dialysis was 110–145/70–85 mm Hg and after dialysis 110–145/70–90 mm Hg. They did not require any antihypertensive drugs, excluding case 8 who was recently introduced to dialysis with some residual kidney function. Severe problems did not occur in our patients over these 6 years excluding blood access infection twice, slipping out of a needle during dialysis with small blood loss once, and drop in blood pressure at the end of dialysis once, which was recovered by her assistant's help.

Our HHD Training and Overnight HHD

Our HHD training program is divided into three parts. Part 1 includes preparation (priming blood lines and dialyzer, and gas purge of dialysis fluid circuit), handling bloodlines, checking vital signs during dialysis, dealing with a dialysis machine and its alarms, teaching the aseptic manipulation, recording data on the dialysis chart. Part 2 includes puncturing a blood access, connecting blood lines to puncture needles, returning blood to the body at the end of dialysis, removing needles and stanching the puncturing parts of blood access, and handling the waste disposal of dialysis. Part 3 is called pre-HHD, which is done in the single room of our clinics, and includes handling a single patient dialysis machine and reverse osmosis system, rinsing a dialysis machine, sampling the blood for laboratory tests, making an inventory of expendable medical supplies including dialysis fluid, heparin, saline, and the final reconfirmation of HHD. What is more, part 3 includes guiding the patient's assistant to flush saline into the needle in order to reduce the high venous pressure and to return blood to the body on emergency and finally teaching both a patient and assistant how to troubleshoot using a troubleshooting procedure list.

The average training duration for HHD was 106 ± 42 days. The shortest was 60 days and longest 198 days. Case 2 underwent his HHD training in another clinic before he came to us. Part 1 was not difficult for all patients. Part 2 was sometimes difficult for them. They needed time to puncture a blood access well. If puncturing was not so difficult for the patients, they did not need more time to clear part 2. These differences among training durations might be caused by the better hand of puncturing and frequency of training times weekly. The frequency of our HHD training was flexible. Some patients came to us 3 times weekly or more, and the others once a week such as on Sunday. Part 3 did not take time because they could move to part 3 after everything regarding HHD training had been approved by us. We did not instruct any additional issues and points for overnight HHD, because performing overnight HHD is similar to doing standard HHD. Some patients moved to overnight HHD slowly starting with once weekly and the others started overnight HHD several days after they had started HHD.

Problems, Difficulties, and Questions

It was not easy for patients to perform HHD at home in the beginning, although they had approval by us to start HHD after being thoroughly

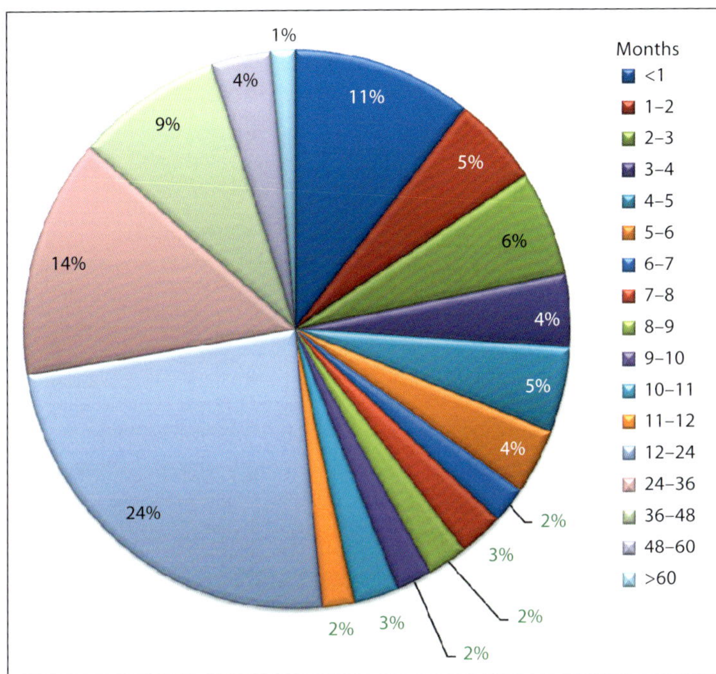

Fig. 1. Our 29 HHD patients, whose duration of HHD was 2.9 ± 2.2 years, called us regarding their HHD. We had 423 calls in total for 6 years. We divided those calls when they called us after their first HHD. Almost half of all calls were done within a year.

trained. If the patients had some questions before or during dialysis, or some problems such as in puncturing a blood access, handling a dialysis machine, machine problems, dialysis fluid, sampling blood for laboratory test, and so on, we strongly asked them to call us. We always advised them to stop their dialysis treatments if some problems occurred during dialysis and it was not restored. Calling us was very important and we received any call at any time. We had 423 calls from our 29 HHD patients whose duration of HHD was 2.9 ± 2.2 years for these 6 years. Although some patients' durations of HHD were shorter than 6 years, it might be interesting to analyze their calls. Figure 1 shows when they called us after their first HHD. Almost half of all calls were done within a year. Their calls decreased year for year. Figure 2 shows the reasons, items, and details of their calls. The most frequent calls concerned machine problems, accounting for 27% of all calls. The second most frequent problems concerned handling machines, accounting for 16% of all calls. The major problems were questions on how to deal with a dialysis machine after their failure in handling it whilst preparing for dialysis. The third most frequent calls concerned puncturing a blood access and blood access itself, accounting for 16% of all calls. Puncturing a blood access is the

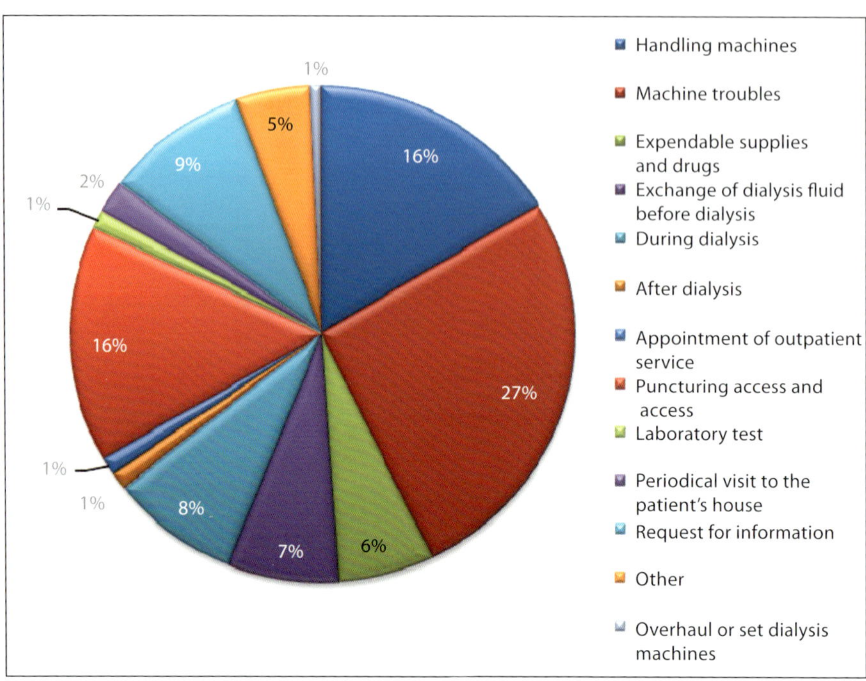

Fig. 2. Our received 432 calls were divided according to their reasons and items. Major troubles were machine problems, handling machines, puncturing a blood access and blood access.

most worrying issue for all, because it cannot be resolved by phone. Some patients came to us and asked us to puncture a blood access as they had failed to do so after they had already started HHD.

Discussion

HHD was started in the USA and England in 1964 [2–4] because patients needed the longer dialysis treatment to maintain their lives and hospitals/institutes did not have enough space, machines, or funding. For example, some 90% of their dialysis patients received overnight HHD 3 times weekly in Seattle Artificial Kidney Center [7] and about 40% of all patients in the USA were on HHD [8] by the early 1970s. Along with an increasing number of dialysis patients, hemodialysis technology, such as blood access, dialysis machine, dialyzer and its membrane, dialysis fluid, blood line, needle, drugs for complications, etc., has improved. Economic and social conditions have also improved in these countries. Such improvements and changes have helped decrease the number of HHD patients. They and new dialysis patients could visit dialysis units for their treatments in

                                    Tanaka · Sakai · Kita · Okamoto · Mikami

the 1980s. Some other reasons why the number of HHD patients was decreasing were the aging of the patients and assistants, newly developed CAPD, and other new technologies for dialysis. In 1997, Buoncristiani et al. [9] reported that daily dialysis was both frequent and efficient, and therefore seemed to be superior to any other form of renal replacement therapy, and Pierratos et al. [10] reported the evidence that high-frequency as well as long-duration hemodialysis provided better clinical outcomes. At that time they could use well-improved hemodialysis systems, the same as we are now using in our dialysis units. For over 10 years, frequent and longer dialysis has been evaluated as having a lot of clinical benefits and overnight HHD is on the return with frequent to daily modes. There are so many studies and reports which have shown multiple benefits of frequent nocturnal hemodialysis compared to conventional 3 times weekly treatments [11–14]. However, Rocco et al. [15] recently reported negative data regarding frequent nocturnal hemodialysis. They did not find a significant effect of nocturnal hemodialysis for either of the co-primary outcomes between conventional hemodialysis (3 times weekly) and nocturnal hemodialysis (6 times weekly). We cannot follow the changes in HHD of those advanced countries or give an objective comment about the reports with our small number of patients and 6 years of experience. However, we can say that our overnight HHD patients are content and enjoy their lives with self-treatment.

When we legally started out HHD program in April 1998 in Japan, many nephrologists and administrators of Japanese hospitals hesitated to introduce HHD. They were afraid of a drop in blood pressure and accidents during dialysis. Furthermore, at the time, reimbursement of HHD was very much lower than that of standard hemodialysis. It then declined in April 2010. The mean reimbursement per month of our overnight HHD patients is now JPY 330,340 ± 3,677, which is comparatively acceptable in comparison with standard hemodialysis. The reimbursement of HHD is mainly split in some disease management fees, which is fixed and JPY 203,050/month in total and the cost of monthly used expendable medical supplies, such as dialyzer, dialysis fluid, heparin, saline, etc. On the other hand, the reimbursement of our 3 times weekly standard dialysis patients in our clinics was JPY 386,090 ± 4,154, which has been on the decline every 2 years. The reimbursement of overnight HHD is basically the same as with daytime HHD.

Conclusion

We have reviewed our HHD program and 8 overnight HHD patients with 6 years' experience. Their general conditions and laboratory data were quite good. Severe problems during overnight HHD did not occur often. We can say that overnight HHD is a safe treatment and our overnight HHD program is suitable for longer and more frequent hemodialysis at home.

References

1   Kolff WJ, Berk HTHJ: The artificial kidney: a dialyser with a great area. Acta Med Scand 1944;117:121–134.
2   Curtis FK, Cole JJ, Fellows BJ, Tyler LL, Scribner BH: Hemodialysis in the home. Trans Am Soc Artif Intern Organs 1965;11: 7–10.
3   Hampers C, Merrill JP, Cameron E: Hemodialysis in the home – a family affair. Trans Am Soc Artif Intern Organs 1965;11: 3–6.
4   Shaldon S: Experience to date with home hemodialysis; in Scribner BH (ed): Proceedings of the Working Conference on Chronic Dialysis. Seattle, University of Washington, 1964, p 66.
5   Baillod R, Comty C, Shaldon S: Overnight haemodialysis in the home. Proc Eur Dial Transpl Assoc 1965;2:99–104.
6   Nakai S, Iseki K, Itami Y, Ogata S, Kazama J, Kimata N, Shigematsu T, Shinoda T, Syoji T, Suzuki K, Taniguchi M, Tsuchida K, Nakamoto H, Nishi H, Hashimoto S, Hasegawa T, Hanafusa N, Hamano T, Fujii N, Masakane I, Marubayashi S, Morita O, Yamagata K, Wakai T, Wada A, Watanabe Y, Tsubakihara Y: An overview of dialysis treatment in Japan as of December 31, 2009. J Jap Soc Dial Ther 2011;44:1–36.
7   Blagg CR, Clark M, Pollard TL, Sawyer TK: A regional program for the treatment of chronic renal failure. Vth International Congress of Nephrology, Mexico City 1972, p 15.
8   Blagg CR: Incidence and prevalence of home dialysis. J Dial 1977;1:475–493.
9   Buoncristiani U, Fagugli R, Quintaliani G, Kulurianu H: Rationale for daily dialysis. Home Hemodial Int 1997;1:12–18.
10 Pierratos A, Ouwendyk M, Francoeur R, Vas S, Raj DSC, Ecclestone A-M, Langos V, Uldall R: Nocturnal hemodialysis: three-year experience. J Am Soc Nephrol 1998;9: 859–868.
11 Ayus JC, Mizani MR, Achinger SG, Thadhani R, Go AS, Lee S: Effects of short daily versus conventional hemodialysis on left ventricular hypertrophy and inflammatory markers: a prospective, controlled study. J Am Soc Nephrol 2005;16:2777–2788.
12 Kundhal K, Pierratos A, Chan CT: Newer paradigms in renal replacement therapy: will they alter cardiovascular outcomes? Cardiol Clin 2005;23:385–391.
13 Komenda P, Chan C, Pauly RP, Levin A, Copland M, Pierratos A, Sood MM, CAN-SLEEP Investigators: CANadian Slow Long Nightly ExtEnded Dialysis Programs. The evaluation of a successful home hemodialysis program: establishing a prospective framework for quality. Clin Nephrol 2009;71: 467–474.
14 Marshall MR, Hawley CM, Kerr PG, Polkinghorne KR, Marshall RJ, Agar JW, McDonald SP: Home hemodialysis and mortality risk in Australian and New Zealand populations. Am J Kidney Dis 2011;58: 782–793.
15 Rocco MV, Lockridge RS Jr, Beck GJ, Eggers PW, Gassman JJ, Greene T, Larive B, Chan CT, Chertow GM, Copland M, Hoy CD, Lindsay RM, Levin NW, Ornt DB, Pierratos A, Pipkin MF, Rajagopalan S, Stokes JB, Unruh ML, Star RA, Kliger AS and the Frequent Hemodialysis Network (FHN) Trial Group: The effects of frequent nocturnal home hemodialysis: the Frequent Hemodialysis Network Nocturnal Trial. Kidney Int 2011;80:1080–1091.

Hiroshi Tanaka
Ashiya Sakairumi Clinic
10-13 Hama-Ashiyacho, Ashiya 659-0054 (Japan)
Tel. +81 797 31 9911
E-Mail tanaka6302@yahoo.co.jp

Suzuki H (ed): Home Dialysis in Japan.
Contrib Nephrol. Basel, Karger, 2012, vol 177, pp 143–150

Practice of Home Hemodialysis in Dialysis Clinic

Kobin Tomita

Tomita Dialysis Clinic, Kusatsu City, Shiga, Japan

Abstract

The number of dialysis patients in Japan was approximately 300,000 at the end of 2010. Among these patients, however, the number of those undergoing home hemodialysis (HHD) was only 279 (<0.1%). It is clear that HHD is a superior treatment to in-center hemodialysis, because of the unlimited frequency and time of HHD, as well as its association with a higher QOL and greater improvement in complications (e.g. hypertension). However, there are still many challenges to be overcome in order to disseminate HHD. It has yet to become widely available, partially because of low-level recognition among dialysis patients and healthcare workers providing dialysis, rather than problems regarding medical technologies and the economy. Of the 16 HHD patients in this center, 10 are practicing overnight hemodialysis, and they are extremely satisfied with its advantages: prolonged treatment yields a better health condition, the dialysis time seems shorter than 1 h by practicing it during hours that include the sleeping time, their complexion becomes as favorable as that of healthy persons, their itchy sensation resolves, they feel as if their physical conditions have returned to a normal level, and their QOL surprisingly increases. Training for HHD is conducted in the dialysis unit along with other patients receiving dialysis treatment (three times a week). Such training lasts for approximately 3 months, during which time patients continue their work. After the initiation of HHD at home, patients and their caregivers can contact our center staff with a cellular phone at any time so they do not need to feel anxious. We hope that many patients will practice HHD in order to resume an active daily life.

It has been more than 10 years since health insurance coverage for home hemodialysis (HHD) became available in 1998 in Japan. At the end of 2010, the number of dialysis patients was 297,126, among whom those undergoing home HHD numbered only 279 [1]. This center began to employ HHD in 2004, and, initially, the procedure was not well organized, and it could be introduced to only one patient or so per year. Currently, however, HHD can be introduced to a few patients annually due to improvement in the technologies. It is clear that HHD is a superior treatment to in-center hemodialysis, because of the unlimited frequency and time of HHD, as well as its association with a higher QOL and greater improvement in complications (e.g. hypertension), but there are still many challenges to be overcome in order to disseminate HHD in Japan. There are some issues for patients, such as anxiety, that they may not be able to master the procedure, anxiety over problems that may occur during dialysis, and much lower insurance points for HHD than in-center dialysis. The biggest issue is, however, probably that not only patients, but also healthcare workers do not fully understand HHD. As frequent and long-term dialyses have been highly evaluated in recent years [2–4], HHD is estimated to rapidly disseminate in Japan under the current insurance system, if it becomes widely recognized. This report introduces the state regarding HHD, which is introduced particularly to outpatients in this center.

Education and Training for HHD

Patients who are undergoing nighttime dialysis in this center visit between 16:00 and 19:00 h to receive treatment for 4–5 h. We describe a male daytime worker undergoing nighttime dialysis three times a week, to whom HHD was introduced. He usually presents to this center after work to undergo dialysis from around 18:00 h. His wife, who is his caregiver, visits this center between 16:30 and 17:00 h to learn about the structure of the dialysis circuit, and dialyzer operation. She subsequently observes the patient's training for vascular puncture, and learns to initiate the procedure with him. She goes home for housework when dialysis is initiated. At 21:45 h, she returns to this center, and learns to discontinue HHD. Finally, at 22:30 h, the patient and his wife go home.

Education and training for HHD are conducted on the dialysis floor instead of a private room, thereby facilitating other patients' observation, which may raise their awareness regarding HHD (fig. 1). Patients and their caregivers receive education from our center staff, mainly nurses and technicians, at each dialysis treatment for 3 months or shorter. Subsequently, physicians determine whether patients and their caregivers can practice HHD at home. For the first week from its initiation at home, the nurses and technicians responsible visit patients in turn to check whether dialyzer operation and vascular puncture are being appropriately conducted. Physicians visit patients once during this period to check for any problems. Because the nurses and technicians responsible use the same cellular phone in turn, it is possible to contact them at any time, therefore patients and their caregivers do not need to feel anxious. If patients are married women and taken care of by their husbands who are company employees, intensive training for HHD is provided on their husbands' days off, such as Saturdays. The patient learns about the structure of

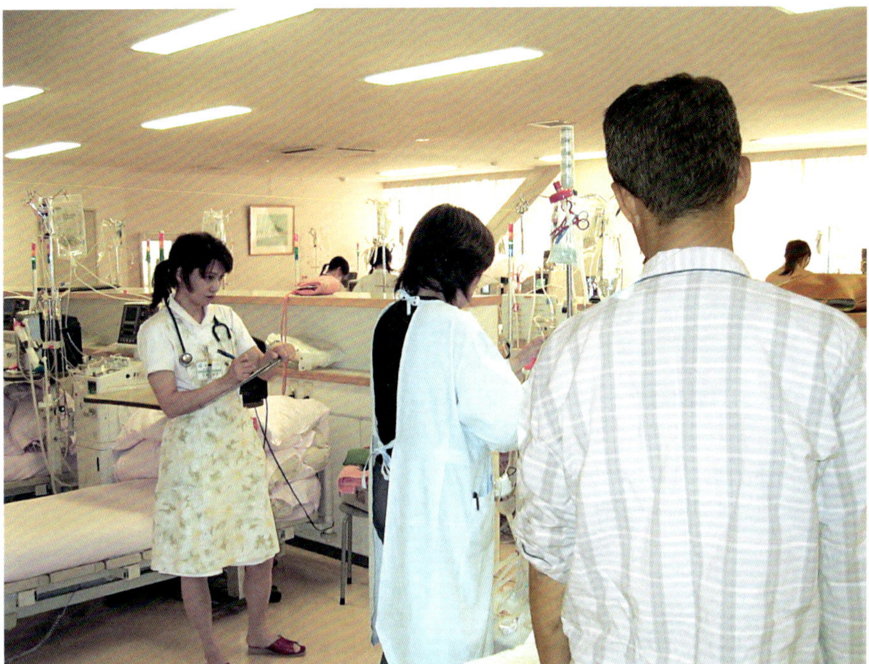

Fig. 1. A nurse instructing a patient and his wife about HHD on the dialysis floor.

the dialysis circuit as well as vascular puncture twice a week, and her husband intensively learns about the dialyzer operation on Saturdays. Thus, the training is designed to conclude within 3 months. After its conclusion, a patient and caregiver take simple written and practical examinations, and, if they pass, HHD can be initiated at home.

In this center, the ages of HHD patients vary considerably, and the oldest patient is a 74-year-old man with diabetes. He has been practicing HHD since the age of 69, when his wife was 67 years old. He saw other patients receiving training for HHD in the dialysis unit and requested his and his wife's participation. It was explained based on their ages that it would be impossible for them to master the dialyzer operation and vascular puncture. However, their participation was allowed by a physician because of their strong requests, and they could eventually master the procedure after approximately 4 months of training. They are now enjoying their lives while working in agriculture. The patient has impaired eyesight due to diabetic retinopathy, and so his wife conducts vascular puncture on his behalf (fig. 2). Our center staff emergently visits the patient once or twice a year to solve puncture-related problems, but they have continued HHD for 5 years without major accidents. This case showed that elderly patients can also master HHD if they are willing to do so, and receive sufficient support from their caregivers.

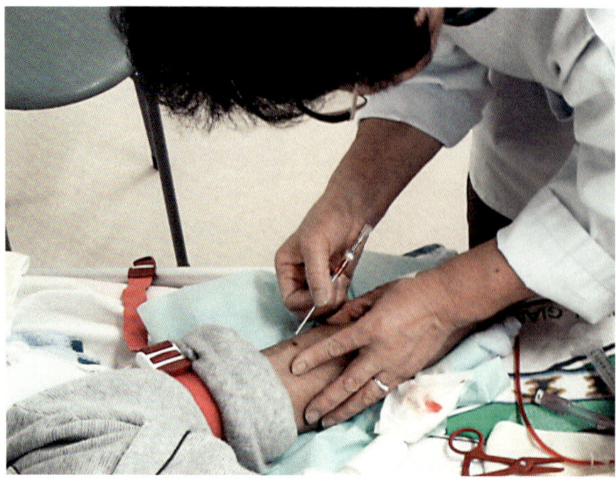

Fig. 2. A 69-year-old patient has impaired eyesight due to diabetic retinopathy, so his wife conducts a vascular puncture on his behalf.

The greatest challenge during the training is vascular puncture for most patients. Buttonhole puncture is common in consideration of fear over pain, but, if this fails, normal puncture may be conducted after the application of xylocaine tape. Of the 16 HHD patients in this center, 12 practice self-puncture, and, for the remaining 4 patients, their caregivers (2 are nurses) conduct puncture. It is described in the 'Home Hemodialysis Management Manual' [5] issued by the Japanese Association of Dialysis Physicians that puncture is only allowed to be performed by patients themselves. In this center, however, caregivers are also allowed to conduct puncture if they are considered to be better at it than patients.

The State Regarding HHD

Of approximately 180 outpatients undergoing dialysis in this center, 16 are practicing HHD. Prior to the initiation of HHD, patients enter into a contract with this center, assuming that they are deemed responsible enough to conduct the procedure. They are also informed that HHD should not be suspended for 2 days or longer. HHD is differently practiced according to each patient's lifestyle (table 1). In addition to its flexibility, such as the availability of daily practices and long-hour practices at night, HHD can resolve an itchy sensation and malaise, for which the degree of patients' satisfaction is much higher for HHD than in-center dialysis.

In this center, dialysis staff regularly hold social gatherings for HHD patients and their caregivers to prevent them from feeling isolated, and promote the

Table 1. Dialysis plan and dose (June 2011)

Case	Sex	Time per treatment h	Weekly frequency	Time per week h	HDP
1 (NHHD)	M	8	4	32	128
2 (NHHD)	M	7	3.5 (every 2 days)	24.5	85.75
3 (NHHD)	M	8	3.5 (every 2 days)	28	98
4	M	4.5	4	18	72
5 (NHHD)	M	7	3.5 (every 2 days)	24.5	85.75
6 (NHHD)	M	7.5	4	30	120
7	F	4.5	3.5 (every 2 days)	15.75	55.13
8	F	4.5	3.5 (every 2 days)	15.75	55.13
9	M	5	3.5 (every 2 days)	17.5	61.25
10	F	5	3.5 (every 2 days)	17.5	61.25
11 (NHHD)	M	8	3.5 (every 2 days)	28	98
12	F	5	3.5 (every 2 days)	17.5	61.25
13 (NHHD)	M	7.5	3.5 (every 2 days)	26.3	91.9
14 (NHHD)	F	7	3.5 (every 2 days)	24.5	85.75
15 (NHHD)	M	7.25	4	29	116
16 (NHHD)	M	6	4	24	96

active exchange of information between them (HHD outpatients in this center have few occasions to meet socially, because they present here for examination only about twice a month). A few years ago, a male patient shifted to nocturnal home hemodialysis (NHHD), which is conducted during hours that include sleeping time, because of his busy work. He stated that his complexion became as favorable as that of a healthy person, his malaise occurring after dialysis resolved, and a normal daytime life could be resumed. This case prompted other patients to initiate NHHD, and the number of those practicing such dialysis gradually increased. Of the 16 HHD patients in this center, 10 are practicing NHHD, and they state that prolonged treatment yields a better health condition, their complexion became as favorable as that of healthy persons, and the time of NHHD seems very short because it is conducted during hours that include sleeping time. Scribner and Oreopoulos [6], who suggested that the use of Kt/V as a dialysis measure is associated with a poor prognosis in dialysis patients, recommend a hemodialysis product (HDP) of 70 or higher as a measure of sufficient dialysis doses. Those 10 patients are showing an HDP of 80 or higher, and 2 of them are showing an HDP exceeding 100 (table 1):

$$\text{HDP} = (\text{dialysis time}) \times (\text{dialysis frequency/week})^2$$

It was clarified that blood pressure (BP) becomes stable to an extent that antihypertensive medications are hardly necessary after each NHHD treatment, and is also likely to remain stable during days when NHHD is not conducted. Due to a dialysis time ranging from 7 to 8 h, a low ultrafiltration rate is achieved, and the interruption of dialysis due to excessive lowering of BP rarely occurs. Patients' caregivers are also satisfied with NHHD, which does not need to be conducted during busy hours for housework. According to Pierratos [7], who conducted a clinical study to evaluate patients practicing daily NHHD, phosphorus (P) was added to dialysis fluids due to the excessive lowering of P values. However, those 10 patients maintain their predialysis P values between approximately 3.5 and 5.5 mg/dl, and NHHD that is practiced twice daily or four times a week does not cause a decrease in serum P values to an extent that the addition of P is required.

HHD is differently practiced according to each patient's lifestyle, and the following advantages were revealed based on a questionnaire survey involving the 16 patients, and their clinical courses after HHD introduction [8]: (1) daily practices and long-hour practices at night are possible; (2) they have more time compared to in-center dialysis patients and can therefore even work overtime; (3) they can spend more time with their family members, and (4) HHD can be practiced in a private room (they can be relaxed, have coffee, or listen to music or watch TV without earphones).

On the other hand, the disadvantages of HHD based on the survey were problems regarding the dialyzer and anxiety over changes in physical condition (e.g. decreased BP) during treatment, but it was clarified that such problems and anxiety can be solved over the phone in most cases. In addition, all HHD patients in this center live within a 30-min drive and hence our center staff can visit them on short notice to solve problems regarding a dialyzer or puncture. In fact, however, such problems are mostly solved over the phone, and our center staff rarely visit HHD patients. If puncture-related problems continuously occur, re-training for vascular puncture may be temporarily provided in this center. Economic burdens may also concern HHD patients. In Japan, medical costs for dialysis are mostly covered by the public insurance system, but HHD-related electricity and water fees need to be individually paid (JPY 7,000–15,000 yen/month). The establishment of a public financial support system is desirable considering that medical costs for HHD are much less expensive than those for in-center dialysis.

The advantages of HHD markedly outnumber those of in-center dialysis in terms of the clinical course. In patients practicing HHD, the levels of substances with small molecular weights (e.g. BUN, Cr, and P) and proteins with small molecular weights (e.g. β_2-microglobulin) decrease. The amount of erythropoiesis-stimulating agents used also decreases due to improved anemia. Before the initiation of HHD, patients were strongly worried that their BP might decrease during dialysis. In fact, however, the interruption of HHD due to excessive lowering of BP has not occurred, and their BPs remain surprisingly stable for days when HHD is not conducted. This tendency is markedly observed particularly in those practicing prolonged dialysis. Of the 16 HHD patients in this center, some have a history of myocardial infarction or ruptured aortic dissecting aneurysm (Stanford type 1), but their clinical courses have been extremely favorable due to a stable BP, and HHD was suggested to possibly promote the inhibition of complications.

Advantages of HHD

When the 16 HHD patients in this center are compared to those undergoing in-center dialysis, the former show greater improvement in BP as well as other values, and resume more active and flexible daily lives because of the availability of dialysis according to individual lifestyles. We believe that HHD is the optimal dialysis treatment which can be provided under the current medical insurance system. In addition, when patients resume their active lives, the level of satisfaction and sense of accomplishment of healthcare workers involved in HHD treatment markedly increase, and they become further motivated for dialysis treatment. Prolonged and more frequent HHD, without its suspension for 2 days or longer, is estimated to increase patients' QOL and consequently improve their prognoses. However, HHD is not available for some patients due to various limitations. We have been employing overnight in-center hemodialysis since September 2011 for patients requesting prolonged dialysis. Currently, 12 patients are undergoing long-time dialysis during hours that include sleeping at our center three times a week, and each treatment continues for 7–8 h from any time between 21:00 and 23:00 h. These patients are highly satisfied with its advantages: malaise occurring after dialysis resolves, it is possible to work during the daytime, and the dialysis time seems extremely short. Therefore, the number of patients undergoing overnight in-center hemodialysis is likely to increase. Healthcare workers are heavily responsible for overnight in-center hemodialysis, but we are going to continue this practice and hope for improved patient prognoses as well as practice of HHD.

Conclusion

Paternalism has been prevalent in Japanese healthcare settings, and, for example, dialysis staff are generally responsible for the entire procedure from vascular puncture to dialysis discontinuation in dialysis care settings. Therefore, many individuals do not attempt to learn HHD for which patients are required to be fully responsible. In this center, a social gathering focused on learning is held for patients and staff twice annually. Dialysis outpatients are also provided with lectures, which are aimed at raising their awareness regarding the advantages of HHD (e.g. high QOL and favorable data), and to report the opinions of

HHD patients: self-management skills improve through HHD, problems during dialysis decrease (e.g. lowering of BP), and favorable prognoses can be expected. We hope that many Japanese dialysis patients, including those in this center, will understand and practice HHD.

References

1 Current State of Chronic Dialysis Treatment in Japan issued by the Japanese Association of Dialysis Physicians, December 31, 2010.
2 Chertow GM, Levin NW, Beck GJ, Depner TA, Eggers PW, et al, FHN Trial Group: In-center hemodialysis six times per week versus three per week. N Engl J Med 2010;363: 2287–2300.
3 Saran R, Bragg-Gresham JL, Levin NW, Twardowski ZJ, Wizemann V, et al: Longer treatment time and slower ultrafiltration in hemodialysis: associations with reduced mortality in the DOPPS. Kidney Int 2006;69: 1222–1228.
4 Kjellstrand CM, Buoncristiani U, Ting G, Traeger J, Piccoli GB, et al: Short daily haemodialysis: survival in 415 patients treated for 1,006 patient-years. Nephrol Dial Transplant 2008;23:3283–3289.
5 Home Hemodialysis Management Manual issued by the Japanese Association of Dialysis Physicians, February 2010.
6 Scribner BH, Oreopoulos DG: The hemodialysis product: a better index of dialysis adequacy than Kt/V. Dial Transplant 2002;31: 13–15.
7 Pierratos A: Nocturnal home haemodialysis: an update on 5-year experience. Nephrol Dial Transplant 1999;14:2835–2840.
8 Tomita K: Current state and problems regarding home hemodialysis. Jpn J Clin Dial 2010;26:177–182.

Kobin Tomita
Tomita Dialysis Clinic
Kusatsu City, Shiga 525–0025 (Japan)
Tel. +81 77 566 0303
E-Mail k-tomita1125@hotmail.co.jp

Suzuki H (ed): Home Dialysis in Japan.
Contrib Nephrol. Basel, Karger, 2012, vol 177, pp 151–160

Perspective of Home Hemodialysis in Japan

Takefumi Narikiyo · Masahiko Nakamoto

Saiseikai Yahata General Hospital, Kidney Center, Kitakyushu, Japan

Abstract

HHD is one of the ESRD therapies that has been established after more than 35 year's experience in Japan. However, only 279 patients were treated with HHD in 2010, which accounts for 0.1% of 297,000 dialysis patients. Long-term HD has been popular in Japanese dialysis units because of the education and enlightenment by some enthusiastic nephrologists who understand the advantage of slow and long dialyses. Following excellent clinical outcomes from Tassin County in France and the DOPPS study has revealed that long and frequent hemodialyses result in good clinical outcomes. These findings have encouraged Japanese nephrologists to promote intensive hemodialysis treatment in their HD units, and HHD has become the focus of dialysis methods. This review describes the training and practical procedures of HHD in Japan. The barriers of HHD use are discussed from patient-related and medical system-related viewpoints.

History of Home Hemodialysis in Japan

In Japan, home hemodialysis (HHD) therapy was started in 1969 by a group in Nagoya. As HHD therapy was accepted as one of the treatments for end-stage renal disease (ESRD) by the public health insurance (reimbursement system) in 1998, the number of HHD patients tended to increase, although only 279 patients were treated with HHD in 2010, which account for 0.1% of the 297,000 dialysis patients in Japan (fig. 1) [1].

HHD is one of the ESRD therapies that was already established with more than 35 years of experience in Japan, although unawareness of HHD therapy in patients and difficulties in securing an assistant (carer) and an increased number of procedures by themselves in home treatment made it a complicated method.

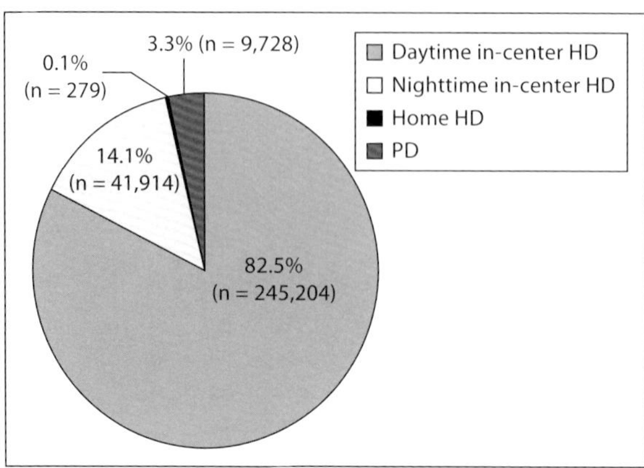

Fig. 1. Dialysis modalities in Japan.

Long-time HD ($\geq$6 h/session, 18 h/week) has been popular in Japanese dialysis units because of the education and enlightenment by some enthusiastic nephrologists who understand the advantages of slow and long dialysis. Excellent clinical outcomes in Tassin, France [2] and the DOPPS study [3] reveal that long and frequent hemodialysis (HD) brings about good clinical outcomes for the patient. Also, in the 1990s a Canadian group created the home daily nocturnal hemodialysis (NHD) program which provided dialysis patients with remarkable and impressive clinical outcomes [4]. These findings encouraged Japanese nephrologists to promote intensive HD treatment in their HD units, and HHD became the focus of dialysis methods. Japanese nephrologists had been struggling to establish an HHD program which has time-flexibility in session schedule planning to extend treatment time and frequency.

Advantages of Long and Frequent HD, and HHD

Advantages of Long and Frequent (Intensive) HD
Table 1 summarizes the clinical benefits of long and frequent HD. Because HHD allows more flexibility for the strategically more demanding schedules of alternate-day or daily HD, HHD is the best HD method by which we can establish long and frequent HD in Japan. There is no risk of blood-transmitted infection, which is the unique advantage of HHD.

Table 2 defines the typical treatment parameters of conventional HD as compared to the intensive HD methods. Intensive HD describes collectively all methods that offer either longer duration or higher frequency of HD compared with CHD (4 h/session, 3 sessions/week), including long (intermittent) HD

Narikiyo · Nakamoto

Table 1. Clinical benefits of intensive HD

Benefits	References
Reduced mortality	2–5
Blood pressure control	6, 7
Left ventricular hypertrophy	8, 9
Arrhythmia	10, 11
Anemia	12, 13
Ca and phosphate control	14, 15
Nutrition	16
Amyloid	17, 18
Depression, mental state	19
Sleep apnea	20
Fertility	21

Table 2. Typical treatment parameters for various HD modalities [data from 23]

Treatment parameters	CHD	LHD	SDHD	SDHD with NSO	NDHD	PD combined
Number of treatments/week	3	3	6	6	5–6	
Treatment time, h	4	8	2–3	2–3.5	7–8	
Interdialytic period, h						
Shortest	44	40	21	20.5	17	
Longest		68	64	45	44.5	41
Blood flow rate, ml/min	400	220	400	400	200	
Dialysate flow rate, ml/min	500	500	800	130	300	

CHD = Conventional hemodialysis; LHD = long hemodialysis; SDHD = short daily hemodialysis; NSO = NxStage System One; NDHD = nocturnal daily hemodialysis.

(intermittent HD (3 sessions/week)) of increased duration, and daily HD (5–7 sessions/week), which may be short daily hemodialysis (SDHD), or daily dialysis of shortened duration, and NHD, or long nightly dialysis [22]. The NxStage System One (NSO) is the only purpose-built machine for HHD on the US market, but is currently not available elsewhere [23].

Dialysis Method in HHD

Many of these techniques can be performed at home. In Japan, long hemodialysis (LHD) (6 h/session, every other day, 3–4 sessions/week) is popular in HHD and the NHD program was put into practice in some HD units several years ago. The average session times in Japan in 2007 were 5.03 h in HHD and

Table 4. Restrictions to use of HHD

Patient-related
- Lack of knowledge about HHD therapy
- Difficulty in securing a cooperative assistant
- Difficulty and fear of self-cannulation
- Problems in preparation and cleaning up
- Additional cost for water, electricity supply, waste management
- ESA injection

Medical system-related
- Cost for training staff and 24 h emergency support
- Lack of public support systems for supplying and waste management
- Dialysis machines

Support and Monitoring for HHD

Planned Hospital Visits
The patient and assistant visit the clinic/hospital once a month and a blood test and chest x-ray is performed to evaluate the patient's physical condition. Technical procedures are evaluated repeatedly in in-center HD treatment at outpatient visits.

Emergency Support
A 24-hour support system for patients' problems is very important for both their safety and confidence in HHD. An HHD patient can call medical staff at the HD room throughout the day and staff are on duty at nighttime to support dialysis therapy. We have examined the frequency and contents of emergency calls: Staff calls from HHD patients are most frequent when starting HHD and just after finishing training. Most of the calls were questions about dialysis machines. Calls decrease 3 months after starting HHD. Visiting cases were very rare. As patients become skilled in HHD therapy, they can sense eventual problems in advance, for example, 'Blood pressure is relatively low recently. And I feel sluggish after dialysis. I would like to change dry weight up to plus 1 kg' and 'Because a typhoon is coming, I will dialyze today'. Sufficient training can make emergency calls infrequent and prevent emergency visits by the staff.

Restrictions of Using HHD

Patient-related and medical system-related HHD restrictions are discussed below (table 4). In spite of its time-flexibility advantages and clinical outcomes, HHD is only a small fraction of ESRD therapies available in Japan. Only 279 patients were treated with HHD in 2010, accounting for 0.1% of the 297,000 dialysis patients in Japan. What restrictions apply to HHD?

Patient-Related Restrictions
(1) *Lack of Knowledge about HHD Therapy.* Our survey revealed that only 30% of 59 HD patients in our HD unit (mean age 63 years; 22 females, 37 males) were willing to try HHD, and 60% refused it. Although they were informed several times about HHD therapy by our staff and almost all of them had enough knowledge of both the method and benefits, most feared eventual emergencies at home. Patients and assistants who undergo HHD training also feel uneasy as to the difficulties and problems of self-medication. Because their fears are obscure in most cases, it is very important to set up a practical problem situation and make both the patient and assistant face a problem solution. Practical case training makes patients/assistants more confident. Lack of information about HHD is a major problem, especially in HD units less experienced with HHD. The Japan Association of Kidney Disease Patients (JAKDP, http://zjk.or.jp/) is taking greater notice of HHD as a favorable dialysis method and spreading information in official journals and at patient meetings nationwide. All medical staff participating in kidney disease healthcare should have sufficient knowledge about HHD. People interested in HHD and contact a nearby dialysis unit where the medical staff cannot provide them with adequate information will be discouraged. The task for nephrologists is to convince the staff and patients to understand the necessity of longer and more frequent dialysis sessions to improve outcomes.

(2) *Difficulty in Securing a Cooperative Assistant.* The carer (assistant) has an indispensable role in HHD treatment for patient safety. In most cases in Japan the carer is either the wife or parent, and spending a great deal of time to train and accompany the HHD patient is a considerable burden for them. The medical staff has to be cautious about the carer's stress and anxiety, and intervene if necessary.

(3) *Difficulty and Fear of Self-Cannulation.* Patients have to puncture their blood access themselves except if the carer is a nurse, medical engineer or medical doctor. Sufficient training can make self-cannulation safe.

(4) *Troubles in Preparation and Cleaning Up.* In-center HD, setting up the blood circuit and dialysis solution, calculation/planning ultrafiltration rate, blood access puncture, and finishing treatment are undertaken by the staff. HHD patients/assistants have to carry out these procedures themselves. It therefore takes extra time in addition to the dialysis session.

(5) *Additional Costs for Water, Electricity Supply and Waste Management.* The public health insurance system in Japan covers the costs of home dialysis machines, water purification equipment, and blood circuit and dialysis fluids. However, it offers no extra incentives for the costs incurred by additional water, electricity and material consumption in HHD, so the patients have to pay such costs themselves.

(6) *ESA Injection.* Patients are not permitted to inject ESA, vitamin D, and iron by themselves at home in Japan. Long and frequent HD with HHD can reduce ESA use, and long-acting ESA administration at the clinic visit once a month is enough to maintain a patient's hemoglobin levels.

Medical System-Related Restrictions

(1) *Costs for Training Staff and a 24-Hour Emergency Support System.* HD units/hospitals promoting HHD programs have to employ additional highly motivated staff for training, maintenance, and a 24-hour emergency call system. The health insurance system has recently increased the payments for education and maintenance fees, but HHD has financial disadvantages compared with in-center HD. Adequate reimbursement for HHD treatment can encourage more HD units to initiate an HHD program. Intensive HD can reduce total medical costs saving on the use of ESA, hospitalization, blood pressure medication, and phosphate control [25, 26]. Therefore, overall, HHD can be a cost-effective option in ESRD treatment. The cost for dialysis material, medicine, and injections varies greatly in all countries. For example, re-usable items including dialyzers are not available in Japan. HHD opinion leaders should re-discuss these medical funding issues and make approaches to the reimbursement organization and government for HHD promotion. Few HD units having an HHD training program prevent patients from starting training, but many dialysis facilities in Japan have recently started an HHD program and applicants can easily access the nearby facility.

(2) *Lack of Public Support Systems for Supplying and Waste Management.* PD companies in Japan have their own supply system for PD solution and deliver and have a 24-hour support call center for patients. No available system exists for HHD burden, HHD maintenance units/hospitals, delivering dialysis materials, solutions and waste management, etc. Because supply systems are very costly, a public system needs to be organized as soon as possible.

(3) *Dialysis Machines.* HHD patients use personal dialysis machines like those for in-center HD. Smaller, less space-occupying, silent, simple purpose-built machines for HHD are required. Some patients have difficulties operating their dialysis machine and setting up the blood circuit. All these problems will eventually be overcome with use of novel HHD technologies.

Perspective of HHD in Japan

To provide ESRD patients with the best clinical outcomes, nephrologists have to apply them long and frequent HD (especially NHD). The practitioners involved in intensive HD are already convinced of the good clinical course and benefits, but a randomized, controlled trial would be required to prove the superiority of intensive HD over CHD.

Narikiyo · Nakamoto

In 2007, the Frequent Hemodialysis Network Trial Group designed a randomized controlled study of NHD versus CHD and published some persuasive results [27, 28]. HHD is an attractive and powerful method to provide patients with long and frequent HD. Pierratos [29] suggested with enthusiasm that daily NHD at home is best for improving the outcomes of patients on dialysis, and in-center nightly HD is an attractive option when HHD is not possible. We have to follow his passion for improvement and advancement, and be fully aware of our responsibility in promoting intensive dialysis. Flexibility in making dialysis schedules and adaptation to the patient's daily life, making modifications according to individual country situations, and harmonious use of public resources are important to establish extensive HD. In a global environment of healthcare accountability and responsibility, it will behoove us to master the knowledge and skills for long and frequent dialysis, to establish the dialysis system including HHD, and to support and advocate for the best care for the dialysis patients throughout their lives.

References

1 Japanese Society for Dialysis Therapy: An overview of dialysis treatment in Japan as of December 31, 2010 (in Japanese) (http://www.jsdt.or.jp/).

2 Laurent G, Charra B: The results of an 8 h thrice weekly haemodialysis schedule. Nephrol Dial Transplant 1998;13(suppl 6): 125–131.

3 Saran R: Longer treatment time and slower ultrafiltration in hemodialysis: associations with reduced mortality in the DOPPS. Kidney Int 2006;69:1222–1228.

4 Pierratos A, Ouwendyk M, Francoeur R, Vas S, Raj DS, Ecclestone AM, Langos V, Uldall R: Nocturnal hemodialysis: three-year experience. J Am Soc Nephrol 1998;9:859–868.

5 Suzuki K, Iseki K, Nakai S, Morita O, Itami Y, Tsubakihara Y: The Committee of Renal Registry, the Japanese Society for Dialysis Treatment. Nihon Toseki Igakkai Zasshi 2010;43:551–559.

6 Charra B, Calemard E, Ruffet M, Chazot C, Terrat JC, Vanel T, Laurent G: Survival as an index of adequacy of dialysis. Kidney Int 1992;41:1286–1291.

7 Shoji T, Tsubakihara Y, Fujii M, Imai E: Hemodialysis-associated hypotension as an independent risk factor for two-year mortality in hemodialysis patients. Kidney Int 2004; 66:1212–1220.

8 Culleton BF, Walsh M, Klarenbach SW, Mortis G, Scott-Douglas N, Quinn RR, et al: Effect of frequent nocturnal hemodialysis vs. conventional hemodialysis on left ventricular mass and quality of life: a randomized controlled trial. JAMA 2007;298:1291–1299.

9 Chan CT, Hanly P, Gabor J, Picton P, Pierratos A, Floras JS: Impact of nocturnal hemodialysis on the variability of heart rate and duration of hypoxemia during sleep. Kidney Int 2004;65:661–665.

10 Bleyer AJ: Sudden and cardiac death rates in hemodialysis patients. Kidney Int 1999;55: 1553–1559.

11 Harada Y, Kawanishi H: Kidney and dialysis supplement HDF treatment, 2001, pp 102–105 (in Japanese).

12 Pierratos A: Daily nocturnal home hemodialysis. Kidney Int 2004;65:1975–1986.

13 Puñal J, Lema LV, Sanhez-Guisande D, Ruano-Ravina A: Clinical effectiveness and quality of life of conventional haemodialysis versus short daily haemodialysis: a systematic review. Nephrol Dial Transplant 2008;23: 2634–2646.

14 Chazot C, Jean G: The advantages and challenges of increasing the duration and frequency of maintenance dialysis sessions. Nat Clin Pract Nephrol 2009;5:34–44.

15 Mucsi I, Pierratos A: Control of serum phosphate without any phosphate binders in patients treated with nocturnal hemodialysis. Kidney Int 1998;53:1399–1404.

16 Pierratos A: Nocturnal home haemodialysis: an update on a 5-year experience. Nephrol Dial Transplant 1999;14:2835–2840.

17 Eloot S, Van Biesen W, Dhondt A, Van de Wynkele H, Glorieux G, Verdonck P, Vanholder R: Impact of hemodialysis duration on the removal of uremic retention solutes. Kidney Int 2008;73:765–770.

18 Raj DS, Pierratos A: Beta-2-microglobulin kinetics in nocturnal haemodialysis. Nephrol Dial Transplant 2000;15:58–64.

19 Jaber BL, Lee Y, Collins AJ, Hull AR, Kraus MA, McCarthy J, Miller BW, Spry L, Finkelstein FO, FREEDOM Study Group: Effect of daily hemodialysis on depressive symptoms and postdialysis recovery time: interim report from the FREEDOM (Following Rehabilitation, Economics and Everyday-Dialysis Outcome Measurements) Study. Am J Kidney Dis 2010;56:531–539.

20 Hanly PJ, Pierratos A: Improvement of sleep apnea in patients with chronic renal failure who undergo nocturnal hemodialysis. N Engl J Med 2001;344:102–107.

21 Barua M, Pierratos A: Successful pregnancies on nocturnal home hemodialysis. Clin J Am Soc Nephrol 2008;3:392–396.

22 Perl J, Chan CT: Home hemodialysis, daily hemodialysis, and nocturnal hemodialysis: Core Curriculum 2009. Am J Kidney Dis 2009;54:1171–1184.

23 Lockridge RS Jr, Moran J: Short daily hemodialysis and nocturnal hemodialysis at home: practical considerations. Semin Dial 2008;21: 49–53.

24 JADP: Manual for home hemodialysis. Japanese Association of Dialysis Physicians, 2010.

25 McFarlane PA, Pierratos A, Redelmeier DA: Cost savings of home nocturnal versus conventional in-center hemodialysis. Kidney Int 2002;62:2216–2222.

26 Komenda P, Copland M, Makwana J, Djurdjev O, Sood MM, Levin A: The cost of starting and maintaining a large home hemodialysis program. Kidney Int 2010;77: 1039–1045.

27 Chertow GM, Levin NW, Beck GJ, Depner TA, Eggers PW, Gassman JJ, et al, FHN Trial Group: In-center hemodialysis six times per week versus three times per week. Frequent Hemodialysis Network Trial Group. N Engl J Med 2010;363:2287–2300.

28 Rocco MV, Lockridge RS Jr, Beck GJ, Eggers PW, Gassman JJ, Greene T, Larive B, et al: The effects of frequent nocturnal home hemodialysis: the Frequent Hemodialysis Network Nocturnal Trial. Kidney Int 2011; 80:1080–1091.

29 Pierratos A: Daily nocturnal hemodialysis – a paradigm shift worthy of disrupting current dialysis practice. Nat Clin Pract Nephrol 2008;4:602–603.

Masahiko Nakamoto
Saiseikai Yahata General Hospital, Kidney Center
5-9-27 Harunomachi, Yahatahigashi-Ku
Kitakyushu City 805–0050 (Japan)
E-Mail nakamoto@med.email.ne.jp

Suzuki H (ed): Home Dialysis in Japan.
Contrib Nephrol. Basel, Karger, 2012, vol 177, pp 161–168

Role of Clinical Engineers in Home Hemodialysis

Naoto Ohhashi[a] · Tsuneo Takenaka[b] · Hitoshi Honda[a] ·
Shintarou Isa[a] · Kazuhito Ishikawa[a] · Kazuya Ohhama[a] ·
Hiromichi Suzuki[b]

[a]Division of Blood Purification Saitama Medical University Hospital and
[b]Department of Nephrology, Saitama Medical University, Saitama, Japan

Abstract
Compared to conventional hemodialysis (HD), home hemodialysis (HHD) enables marked increases in HD duration and frequency. Better clinical outcomes have been reported for HHD, including improvements in patient survival and their quality of life. However, statistical analysis by the Japanese Society for Dialysis Therapy in 2010 revealed that only 0.1% of the end-stage renal disease patients received HHD in Japan. In our hospital, clinical engineers as well as doctors and nurses have resolutely been working towards the education, maintenance and management of HHD. More than 30 patients have successfully and safely started HHD within the last 3 years. To carry out HHD, a certain amount of knowledge is required to understand the principles of dialysis and clinical engineering and how to use HD devices. About 50% of the problems during HHD were related to HD devices. Thus, we feel that it is essential to extend HHD so that clinical engineers can systematically structure and support HHD.

Compared to conventional hemodialysis (HD), home hemodialysis (HHD) enables marked increases in HD duration and frequency. Better clinical outcomes have reported for HHD, including improvements in patient survival and their quality of life [1–4]. However, a statistical analysis by the Japanese Society for Dialysis Therapy in 2010 revealed that only 0.1% of the end-stage renal disease patients received HHD in Japan [5]. In our hospital, we started HHD in 1999. Until 2010, 52 patients had been started on HHD. HHD is an excellent choice of treatment among many renal replacement treatments especially when compared to conventional HD, because HHD improves patient survival and their quality of life greatly through increments of dialysis doses [6–8]. From the beginning to the end of each HHD session, all procedures have to be done solely by the patient and the helper (usually a family member). We educate and train the patients themselves and their helpers (family), who have never touched HD devices nor done any medical practice, about medical commonsense as well as the HD procedure to perform HD safely and easily at home. Regarding equipment, HHD needs various devices including a personal HD monitor and a personal reverse osmosis (RO) device. We regularly diagnose the devices and manage all problems even after starting HHD. Thus, clinical engineers seem to be required to participate in the education of patients from the start and in building up a supporting system for regular checks and troubleshooting management. In this section we report the current status of HHD in our hospital and the role of clinical engineers in HHD.

Education and Coaching

In our hospital it takes on average 3 months to teach HHD when the patient visits us three times a week for training. However, patient backgrounds are diverse. Some patients start renal replacement treatment with HHD first while others have experienced years of conventional HD. We make up an educational schedule for each patient with different approaches, taking patient age and intelligence into consideration (fig. 1). However, this schedule is tentative and mainly used to guide the progress of education. This schedule is tailor-made for each patient according to the progress of understanding and practice of HD procedures. Education, especially for practice of HD priming and shunt puncture, is carried out using a video manual and paper-based manual. Previously, we used only a paper-based manual for education of the HD procedure. However, it became apparent through educating many patients that it is difficult for the patients to understand the actual movement using the paper-based manual only. Thus, we made a video manual, making the patient's understanding of the HD procedure deeper and easier by both the reading procedure itself in the paper-based manual and seeing its movement in the video manual. Furthermore, both paper-based and video manuals have chapters to guide emergent responses to problems during HD. This education makes it easy for the patient to see the condition and respond properly if problems arise. There are big differences between conventional HD and HHD regarding HD efficiency and dietary restriction. Thus, the education on knowledge of HD was mainly performed during HD sessions [9].

As mentioned, we educate each patient differently according to his/her background. In our hospital, we do the HHD training in the initial period of education like a teacher. In the middle of the education period, we change the education style to coaching. We respect and increase the patient's subjective activity to manage themselves by supporting and assessing the current status of their progress. Clinical engineers educate mainly about medical engineering

    Ohhashi · Takenaka · Honda · Isa · Ishikawa · Ohhama · Suzuki

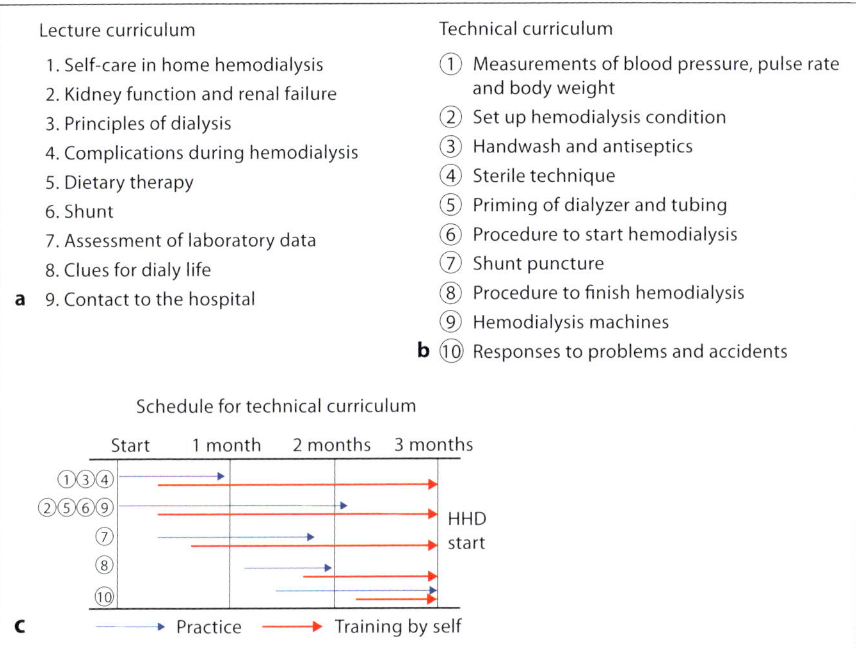

Fig. 1. Curriculum for lecture (**a**), technique (**b**) and its tentative schedule (**c**).

elements including the principles of the HD device, the procedure and the RO machine. We also instruct the patient and the helper about troubleshooting procedures.

Administration of HD Equipment

Pre-HHD Visit

To perform HHD, it is necessary to determine where to place the HD equipment and store the materials required for HD. If needed, the patient is asked to re-arrange their home for draining tubes and power volume in order to obtain adequate water and electrical power. We visit the patient at home before administrating HHD to ascertain their lifestyle, the circumstances in their home and power status. We support the patient to make their home situation suitable for HHD, based on a pre-HHD visit and by taking their lifestyle into consideration.

Transfer of HD Apparatus

As shown in figure 2, we use a personal HD monitor (DBB-27; Nikkiso Co. Ltd) and personal RO equipment (MH-500CX; Japan Water System Co. Ltd)

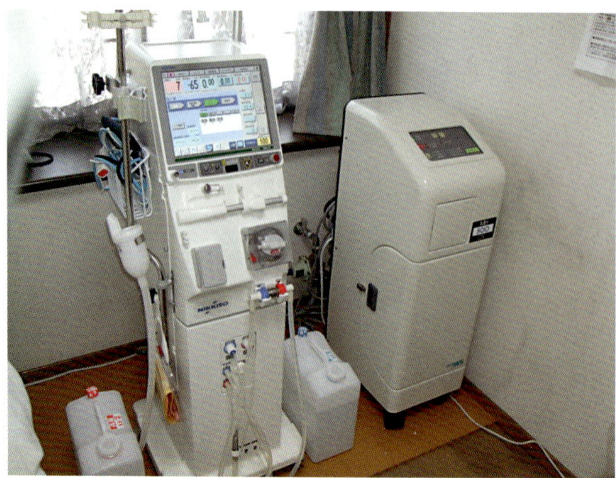

Fig. 2. Transfer and placement of HD apparatus.

for HHD. At the time of allocation of HD apparatus, we appropriately place them in the patient room, run a test drive, make adjustments for dialysate concentrations and set up a timer for sterilization of the HD devices according to the patient's schedule and lifestyle. Thereafter, the patient and helper themselves will start the first session of HHD under our supervision. If we do not come across any problems regarding the patient procedure and equipment, it will be the end of the transfer [10].

Regular Visits
We regularly visit the patient at home once every 3 months to check the HD equipment for any deformities and its running status, and also exchange the consuming apparatus. The RO device is diagnosed regarding its pressure, water volume, and quality. We also check drainage and whether there any water leaks from the tubing, and make a report about findings of the above points. In addition to the hospital staff, staff from the makers of the HD equipment company also visit to maintain and check the equipment. We bring back the original reports to the hospital and load them on an electric medical record with a PDF file, and give the patient a copy of the reports to file them for their own record. In this way we are able to share and check the information of previous records for HD equipment with the patient, hospital staff and company staff. When we visit, we try to resolve any problems concerning technical procedures including shunt puncture by re-explaining and ascertaining the procedure, in addition to equipment diagnosis. We have also started to re-train patients about equipment problems related to power failure after earthquakes [11].

In November 2009, the Japanese Society of Dialysis Therapy proposed the guideline for purification of dialysate version 1.06. In addition to hospitals, it

Ohhashi·Takenaka·Honda·Isa·Ishikawa·Ohhama·Suzuki

is important to obtain purified dialysate for patients on HHD. At the time of a regular visit, we measure two samples for this purpose – one from a sampling port of the personal RO device and the other from dialyzer coupling port of the personal HD monitor. The samples are put into plastic tubes, taken back to the hospital, and used for of endotoxin measurements (Toxinometer Mini) and bacterial culture (surface plate method). All values are maintained below the recommendation by the guideline: endotoxin concentrations of RO water and dialysate <0.01 and <0.001 EU/ml and bacterial count for RO water and dialysate, 5 and 1 CFU/ml, respectively [12, 13].

Problems

Responses to Problems
(a) *By phone (primary response):* Medical staff immediately respond to patients' phone calls with regard to problems that cannot be managed by patients themselves, and instruct them how to resolve the problems.

(b) *Temporal visit (secondary visit):* When the problem is not resolved on the phone (mainly due to machinery troubles), we make a special home visit to perform a maintenance service and fix the equipment.

Content of Troubles
It is important to respond to any problems properly because the patient and the helper have to start and finish HHD safely and easily in the absence of medical staff. We have analyzed previous problems by classifying them into categories such as those related to medical condition (blood pressure drop, etc.), technical procedure (failure to puncture shunt, etc.), environment (drainage overflow, etc.) and devices. We have also revised the educational manuals for patients to respond to common problems during HHD. Thus, the statistics showed that almost half of all the problems were related to HD devices that cannot be fixed by the patient him/herself (fig. 3). However, the number of problems related to the medical condition, technical procedure and environment were relatively small, probably because the patients were able to correct the problems by themselves without calling us. When problems with the device occur, the patient may need to stop HHD temporarily if we are unable to contact the company staff to fix the patient's device [14].

Administration of HD Materials

Dialyzers and the Other Materials Required
The patients request the number of HD materials including dialyzers, needles and syringe once a month to the company directly. The patient also visits the hospital once a month to see a doctor for follow-up, adjusting dry weight and

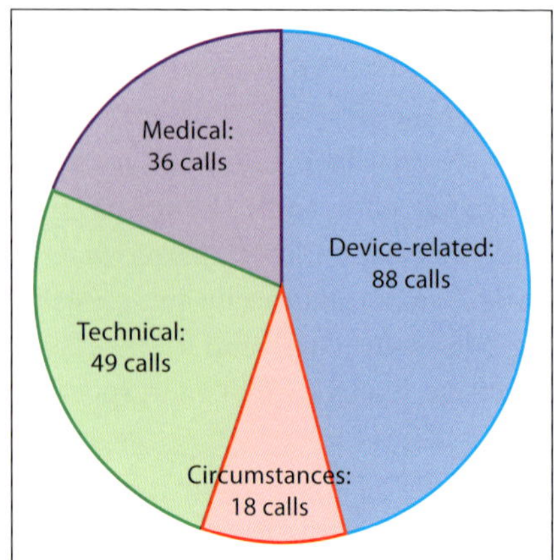

Fig. 3. Numbers of trouble calls from 2001 to 2009 (n = 30).

getting prescriptions such as dialysate, anticoagulant and saline. The pharmacy directly delivers drugs to their home. Every month we obtain documents related to the supply from the company to administer HD materials and HHD itself.

Medical Refuse
Home medical refuse is categorized as general refuse according to the law regarding waste. However, most local governments reject the acceptance of home medical waste. In our hospital we supply patients with boxes to collect medical waste which at the time of their monthly visit they bring with them to the hospital. Although all patients on HHD are officially recognized as being physically handicapped by the Japanese government, they still have to bring two or three boxes each weighing around 20 kg to the hospital at every regular visit. We hope that the local government understands this problem and can make a move to lessen the burden on the patients. If this is not possible, HHD may not prevail in Japan.

Perspectives

It is not easy for the patient and helper to understand medical commonsense such as blood pressure regulation, HD principles, technical issues (shunt puncture) and clinical engineering knowledge on how to handle the machine. Whilst passing on HD knowledge and training patients to master HD techniques, it is important to increase the patient's ability to judge the situation as well as the independence towards their own HD therapy. In other words, it is of paramount importance to have a good and credible relationship between the patient and us. Such a relationship allows the patient to raise questions in addition to us being able to ask the patient questions.

     Ohhashi · Takenaka · Honda · Isa · Ishikawa · Ohhama · Suzuki

It is important to support the patients to make the circumstances in their home suitable for HHD with suggestions for places where to store HD materials and to set up HD machines. We maintain the purity of dialysate by regular assessment of RO water and dialysate, and respond to changes in temperature as well as differences in quality of original water (some houses were supplied with well water). With the administration of HD machines at home, one has to consider the influence of diverse circumstances around the machine and differences in consumption and/or abrasion of parts due to variations of HD duration and frequency. We can say that to prevent machine accidents, the exchange of consuming apparatus and a regular check-up of the each machine should be done very timely according to previous records. To provide the situations for the patient to continue HHD without interruption, we cooperate with company staff to respond quickly to any problems. To maintain better HHD with safety and ease, the doctors, nurses, clinical engineers and company work together as a team for the patient.

Conclusion

Treatment at home is becoming more important to improve the quality of life of patients and their family because of the increasing number of elderly people in general and government policies to cut medical expenses. Recently, new medical devices and equipment for home treatment have been developed. Regarding HHD, various companies have developed small convenient machines, particularly for HHD. However, it is still necessary to administer and maintain medical machines even though safer excellent HHD devices are being developed. However, the role of clinical engineers in HHD as well as home treatment has not been established. In the future we will make every effort to get the government to reimburse the administration of HHD machines and home visits by clinical engineers, similar to home visits by doctors or nurses and visiting occupational and physical therapists. We hope that there will come a time for clinical engineers to resolutely contribute to home treatment as the experts of medical machinery.

References

1 Saito A: Why do patients do home hemodialysis? Merits of home hemodialysis. Dial Front Med Rev Co 2004;14:63.
2 Pierratos A: Daily nocturnal hemodialysis – a paradigm shift worthy of disrupting current dialysis practice. Nat Clin Pract Nephrol 2008;4:602–603.
3 Hanly P: Sleep disorders and home dialysis. Adv Chronic Kidney Dis 2009;16:179–188.
4 Culleton BF, Walsh M, Klarenbach SW, et al: Effect of frequent nocturnal hemodialysis vs. conventional hemodialysis on left ventricular mass and quality of life: a randomized controlled trial. JAMA 2007;298:1291–1299.

  5 Suzuki H: Current status of home hemodi-
    alysis and its problems: clinical engineering
    (in Japanese). Clin Eng Mutual Aid Assoc
    2011;22.
  6 Imada A: Dialysis efficiency suited for home
    hemodialysis, quality of life and survival.
    Clinical dialysis. Japan Medical Center
    2007;23:27–32.
  7 Chertow GW, Levin NW, Beck GJ, et al:
    In-center hemodialysis six times per week
    versus three times per week. N Engl J Med
    2010;363:2287–2300.
  8 Pauly RP, Gill JS, Rose CL, et al: Survival
    among nocturnal home hemodialysis
    patients compared to kidney transplant
    recipients. Nephrol Dial Transplant
    2009;24:2915–2919.
  9 Kjellstrand CM, Buoncristiani U, Ting G,
    et al: Short daily hemodialysis: survival in
    415 patients treated for 1,006 patient-years.
    Nephrol Dial Transplant 2008;23:3283–3289.
 10 Tanaka S: Home hemodialysis machines.
    Clinical dialysis. Japan Medical Center
    2007;23:61–68.
 11 Ohama K, et al: Clinical engineers who
    support stable home hemodialysis with its
    smooth introduction. Clin Eng Mutual Aid
    Assoc 2010;21.
 12 Japanese Society of Clinical Engineers
    Dialysate Working Group: Guideline for
    Purification of Dialysate Version1.06.
 13 Masakane I: Clinical effects of endotoxin-
    free dialysate. Hemodial Endotox 2002;
    49–59.
 14 Ogawa K, et al: Troubles during home hemo-
    dialysis. Clinical dialysis. Japan Medical
    Center 2007;23.

Hiromichi Suzuki, MD, PhD
Department of Nephrology, Saitama Medical University
38 Moroyama-machi, Iruma-gun
Saitama 350-0495 (Japan)
Tel. +81 49276 1620, E-Mail iromichi@saitama-med.ac.jp

    Ohhashi · Takenaka · Honda · Isa · Ishikawa · Ohhama · Suzuki

Suzuki H (ed): Home Dialysis in Japan.
Contrib Nephrol. Basel, Karger, 2012, vol 177, pp 169–177

Daily Hemodialysis Improves Uremia-Associated Clinical Parameters in the Short Term

Eriko Kojima · Hitoshi Hoshi · Yusuke Watanabe · Tsuneo Takenaka · Hiromichi Suzuki

Kidney Disease Center, Saitama Medical University, Department of Nephrology, Saitama Medical University, Saitama, Japan

Abstract

Observational studies suggest that home hemodialysis (HHD) is associated with improvements in several important clinical parameters. These include better control of blood pressure, reductions in left ventricular hypertrophy, calcium-phosphate production, improved nutritional status and enhanced health-related quality of life. In Japan, many case reports and studies of small series of patients treated with HHD have been published mainly in Japanese. The current study was to describe the short-term effects in patients starting HHD at the Kidney Disease Center, Saitama Medical University. This study represents a comprehensive evaluation of the benefits of switching patients from conventional in-center hemodialysis to HHD in Japan. The pertinent findings are as follows: an improvement in blood pressure control paralleled with a reduction in antihypertensive pharmacotherapy, an improvement in serum albumin and hemoglobin levels, and a simultaneous reduction in erythropoietin-stimulating agent, calcium and phosphate levels. In conclusion, our study confirms that selected patients may benefit from HHD which offers an attractive treatment alternative and improvements provided by HHD might ultimately have an impact on patient survival.

Home hemodialysis (HHD) started in Japan in 1961 [1]. Today however, the predominant renal replacement therapy is by in-center dialysis and relevant numbers of patients treated with HHD are reported to be less than 300 compared to nearly 300,000 patients treated with hemodialysis (HD). This is probably due mainly to medical and social reasons. The end-stage renal disease (ESRD) population is now older with a higher fraction of diabetic and polymorbid, disabled patients [2]. In addition, more for-profit units were established which traditionally do not encourage HHD. The advantages of frequent HHD therapy over conventional HD were first reported in the 1960s [3, 4]. Increased dialysis frequency results in more efficient removal of uremic toxins. Observational studies suggest that HHD is associated with improvements in several important clinical parameters. These include better control of blood pressure, reductions in left ventricular hypertrophy (LVH), calcium-phosphate production, improved nutritional status and enhanced health-related quality of life [5–9]. Besides, it has long been recognized that HHD is associated with better patient survival than facility-based HD even with <12 h/week of the conventional dialysis regimen [10–12]. In Japan, many case reports and studies on small series of patients treated with HHD have been published mainly in Japanese. The aim of the current study was to describe the short-term effects of HHD in patients starting HHD at the Kidney Disease Center, Saitama Medical University.

Materials and Methods

This is an observational cohort study with retrospectively collected data. Approval for this study was obtained from the institutional research ethics board. Data on patient demographics such as age, sex, etiology of ESRD and co-morbid conditions were collected from a computerized clinical database. These parameters included the duration and period of ESRD prior to the initiation of HHD. HHD can be performed at home and administered using Nikkiso DBB-27 (Nikkiso Co., Tokyo, Japan) with a water treatment system MH-500CX (Japan Water System Co., Tokyo, Japan). Typical blood flows were 200 ml/min. Sessions varied in length from 3 to 5 h and were performed on an average of 6 times/week. Each patient underwent training on the use of the home dialysis machine for at least 3 months.

Data Collection
Multiple surrogate parameters of known dialysis-associated morbidities were assessed: (1) Dialysis efficacy (creatinine, dry weight). (2) Blood pressure (pre- and postdialytic systolic and diastolic blood pressures, antihypertensive drugs). (3) Nutrition and inflammation (albumin, body mass index). (4) Bone metabolism (calcium, phosphate, intact parathyroid hormone, phosphate-binding pharmacotherapy). (5) Erythropoiesis (hemoglobin, need of erythropoietin-stimulating agent (ESA), need for iron substitution therapy). (6) Echocardiograms of the patients were recorded in the week before the start of treatment and at 6 months after the start of HHD. The measurements included the end-diastole diameter of the left ventricular chamber, the interventricular septum thickness, and the thickness of the left ventricular posterior wall. The left ventricular mass index was calculated from the above measurements according to Devereux and Reichek [13].

All participants were switched from their conventional HD (3 × 4–5 h/week) to the intensified short HHD regimen (6 × 3–5 h/week). During the following 6 months, quarterly follow-up visits were conducted, and all above-mentioned parameters were re-evaluated.

　　　　　　　　　　　　　　　　　　　Kojima · Hoshi · Watanabe · Takenaka · Suzuki

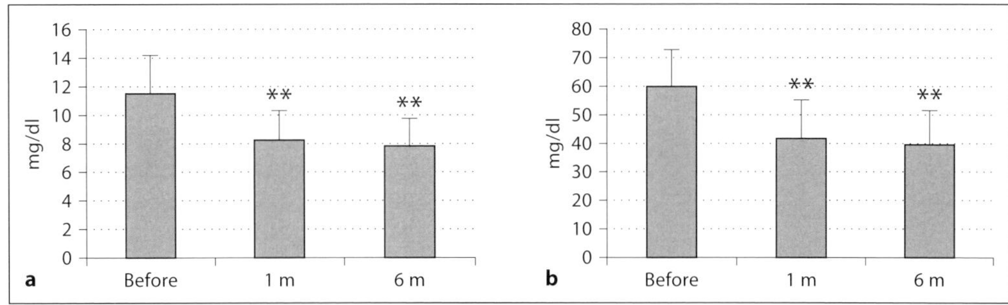

Fig. 1. a Changes in serum creatinine. HHD produced a significant decrease in serum creatinine at 1 and 6 months. **p < 0.01. **b** Changes in blood urea nitrogen. HHD produced a significant decrease in blood urea nitrogen at 1 and 6 months. **p < 0.01.

Statistical Analysis
Values are expressed as mean ± SD. Parameters during the follow-up (baseline (BL) and 6 months) were compared by a nonparametric Friedman's test for paired variables. A p value <0.05 was considered statistically significant.

Results

The mean age of the 54 study participants (46 men, 8 women) was 49.2 ± 10 years, with a dialysis period of 4.0 ± 5.3 years. Underlying renal diseases were as follows: chronic glomerulonephritis 23, diabetes mellitus 11, nephrosclerosis 6, and others 2. Dry weight significantly increased to 101.9 ± 3.9% compared with BL (p = 0.0016).

Blood Pressure and Antihypertensive Drugs. The predialytic systolic blood pressure declined during the study period (BL: 146.2 ± 16.5; 6 months: 124.3 ± 16.0 mm Hg; p < 0.001) but without changes in diastolic blood pressure. At the same time, the number and doses of antihypertensive drugs were reduced (not statistically evaluated).

Serum Creatinine and Blood Urea Nitrogen. HHD reduced the levels of serum creatinine (BL: 11.6 ± 2.5; 6 months: 7.7 ± 1.9 mg/dl; p < 0.00001) and blood urea nitrogen (BL: 59.8 ± 1.3; 6 months: 39.2 ± 11.5 mg/dl; p < 0.00001) (fig. 1a, b).

Serum Albumin and Total Cholesterol. HHD led to marked improvement of the levels of serum albumin (BL: 3.8 ± 0.5; 6 months: 4.1± 0.4 mg/dl; p < 0.005). However, the levels of total cholesterol increased but lacked significance (BL: 157.2 ± 34.2; 6 months: 178.9 ± 37.9 mg/dl) (fig. 2a, b).

Changes in Bone Metabolism. After starting the HHD, serum calcium levels (BL: 9.1 ± 1.1; 6 months: 9.4 ± 0.7 mg/dl) increased but without significance, while serum phosphate levels declined significantly (BL: 5.5 ± 1.5; 6 months: 4.7 ± 1.3 mg/dl; p = 0.025). The amount of phosphate-binding

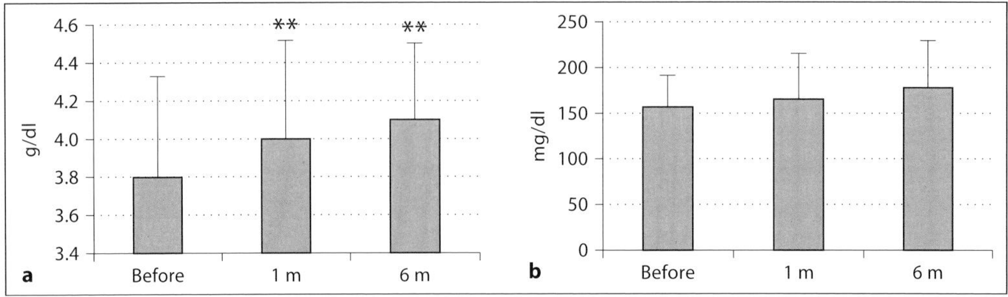

Fig. 2. a Changes in serum albumin. Serum albumin increased significantly at 1 and 6 months after the start of HHD. ****p < 0.01. b** Changes in total cholesterol. Total cholesterol increased at 6 months after the start of HHD, however it lacked significance.

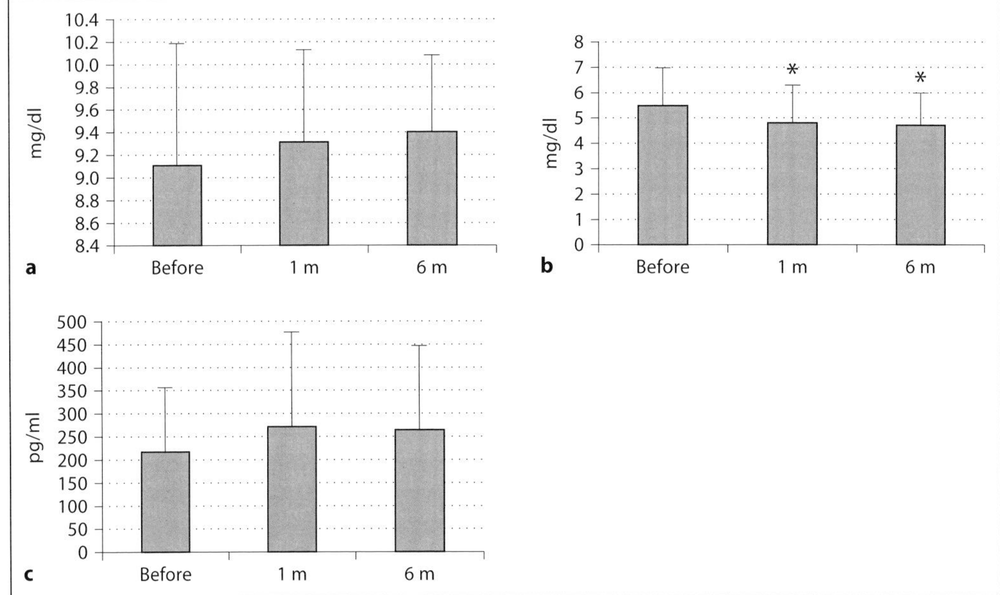

Fig. 3. a, b Changes in serum calcium and phosphate. The levels of serum calcium at 6 months after the start of HHD did not change but those of serum phosphate decreased significantly. *p < 0.05. **c** Changes in plasma intact parathyroid hormone. Plasma intact parathyroid hormone did not show any significant changes during 6 months after the start of HHD.

pharmacotherapy did not change (data are not shown). Intact parathyroid hormone levels increased without significance (BL: 218 ± 137; 6 months: 263 ± 183 pg/ml) (fig. 3a–c)

Hemoglobin Levels Increased Despite a Reduction in ESAs. HHD had no changes in hemoglobin levels (BL: 10.3 ± 0.9; 6 months: 10.4 ± 1.9 g/dl).

Kojima · Hoshi · Watanabe · Takenaka · Suzuki

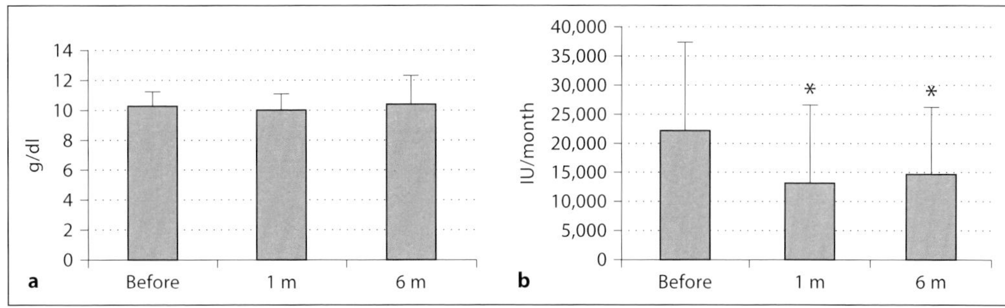

Fig. 4. a, b Changes in hemoglobin and ESA doses. The levels of hemoglobin at 6 months after the start of HHD did not change, however the ESA doses significantly decreased. *p < 0.05.

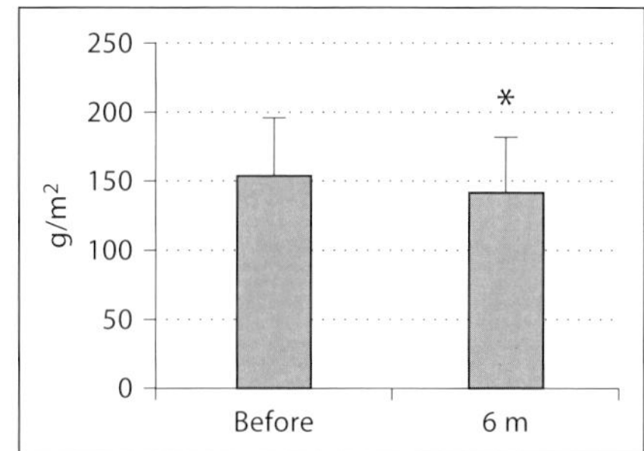

Fig. 5. Changes in left ventricular mass index. LV mass index was significantly reduced at 6 months after the start of HHD. *p < 0.05.

Additionally, the need for ESAs fell significantly (BL: 22,166 ± 15,290; 6 months: 14,555 ± 11,648 IU; p < 0.01) (fig. 4a, b).

Changes in Left Ventricular Hypertrophy. HHD led to a significant reduction in left ventricular mass index (BL: 153.4 ± 42.0; 6 months: 141.4 ± 39.0 g/m²; p < 0.03) (fig. 5).

Discussion

This study represents a comprehensive evaluation of the benefits of switching patients from conventional in-center HD to HHD in Japan. The pertinent findings are as follows: an improvement in blood pressure control paralleled with a reduction in antihypertensive pharmacotherapy, an improvement in serum albumin and hemoglobin levels, and simultaneous reductions in ESAs, calcium and phosphate levels.

Suri et al. [14] published a systematic review of daily HD in 2006. After screening more than 800 citations, 233 full-text articles were reviewed in detail. Of these, only 25 met the inclusion criteria: 5 or more adult patients, follow-up of at least 3 months, dialysis prescribed for 1.5–3 h for 5–7 days/week, and published after 1989. A systematic review of these 25 publications showed consistently improved blood pressure control and reduced LVH. However, the effects of daily HD on quality of life, anemia, phosphorus control and nutritional status were inconsistent.

There is general agreement that systolic, diastolic and mean arterial blood pressures are significantly improved in HHD with a simultaneous reduction in antihypertensive medication requirement [15–18]. This optimal blood pressure control has been associated with regression of left ventricular mass index and improvement according to Culleton et al. [19] in the only randomized controlled trial of nocturnal vs. conventional hours dialysis. Moreover, in 2010 the FHN (Frequent Hemodialysis Network) trial group demonstrated that frequent HD, as compared with conventional HD, was associated with favorable results with respect to the composite outcomes of death or change in left ventricular mass and death or change in a physical-health composite score. It is well known that elevated arterial pressure may be caused by either extracellular volume expansion and/or increased total peripheral resistance [20]. Volume overload is usually attributed to sodium and water retention, whereas pressure overload is linked to increased peripheral resistance and increased arterial stiffness. Chan [21] reported in a retrospective review that 75% of HHD patients had normal blood pressure values without the concomitant use of antihypertensive agents. Fagugli et al. [17] reported in their crossover prospective study that HHD improved blood pressure control and decreased antihypertensive requirements. Both groups measured the change in extracellular fluid content and attributed the blood pressure-lowering effect to a decrease in extracellular fluid volume.

In ESRD patients, LVH is common, and has been shown to be an independent predictor of cardiovascular disease events and survival [22, 23]. Although progression of LVH appears to be the norm in dialysis patients [24], regression of LVH can occur and is associated with improved outcomes (FHN). The mechanisms responsible for this improvement in LVH are uncertain but likely multifactorial. Conceivably, better control of extracellular fluid volume leads to beneficial changes in LVH and blood pressure. In patients on HD, consistently high weight gain between dialysis sessions may induce LVH and other adverse effects [25–27]; a lower weight gain between frequent HHD sessions may be responsible for some improvement of LVH.

A large contributing factor to the increased cardiovascular risk in dialysis patients is vascular calcification and it is well recognized that high calcium, phosphate, and the product of calcium × phosphate are all independent risk factors for cardiovascular events in this patient population [28–30]. It has clearly been shown that superior phosphate control is achieved with nocturnal HD [15, 31]. Conversely, phosphate control is less efficient with short-daily HD [32]. Phosphorus removal in short daily HD sessions is primarily dependent on

     Kojima · Hoshi · Watanabe · Takenaka · Suzuki

the predialysis phosphorus concentration with the amount removed in a week largely depending on session length and frequency of sessions. In addition to duration and frequency, dietary protein and phosphorus intake are important to remember in light of the often conflicting results of short daily HD with regard to phosphorus control and need for phosphorus binders.

A recent systematic review of daily HD concluded that short daily HD had no effect on phosphate control with six of eight studies reporting no significant changes in serum phosphate or phosphate binder dose [14]. However, of the six studies lacking statistical improvement, three showed trends towards lower serum phosphorus levels or phosphate binder use. These three studies used longer treatment sessions and/or more treatments per week than the remaining three studies, which supported the importance of both dialysis frequency and overall treatment time. A study by Ayus et al. [33] demonstrated a significant lowering of serum phosphorus and found that improved phosphorus level was an independent predictor of reduction in LVH.

Contrary to Rao et al. [6], we observed no changes in hemoglobin levels with a reduction in the need for ESAs. In the London/Ontario study, these changes were only of borderline significance, but in our study hemoglobin levels had already increased before the start of HHD and the need for ESAs decreased by 15% in 6 months of intensified HD.

Lastly, it is well known that malnutrition and inflammation impact HD patient survival. Many investigators have shown that serum albumin levels are depressed in maintenance HD patients who manifest other signs of malnutrition [34–36]. In addition, serum albumin levels usually improve as nutrition repletion is accomplished [37].

We are aware that the sample size of our cohort was small, as well as the limited time of the follow-up to 6 months. This obviously restricts the strength of our conclusions. These limitations merely allow for the evaluation of surrogate end-points instead of cardiovascular events. Secondly, the in-center HD and HHD results were not compared. Our study has confirmed that selected patients may benefit from HHD and HHD offers an attractive treatment alternative, and improvements provided by HHD might ultimately have an impact on patient survival.

References

1 Nose Y: Home hemodialysis: a crazy idea in 1963: a memoir. ASAIO J 2000;46:13–7.
2 Nakai S, Suzuki K, Masakane I, Wada A, Itami N, Ogata S, et al: Overview of regular dialysis treatment in Japan as of 31 December 2008. Ther Apher Dial 2010;14: 505–40.
3 DePalma JR, Pecker EA, Gordon A, Maxwell MH: A new compact automatic home hemodialysis system. Trans Am Soc Artif Intern Organs 1968;14:152–159.

4 Sweatman AJ, Baillod RA, Moorhead JF: Comparison of home dialysis and other treatments for chronic renal failure. Practitioner 1974;212:56–66.

5 Fagugli RM, Reboldi G, Quintaliani G, Pasini P, Ciao G, Cicconi B, et al: Short daily hemodialysis: blood pressure control and left ventricular mass reduction in hypertensive hemodialysis patients. Am J Kidney Dis 2001;38:371–376.

6 Rao M, Muirhead N, Klarenbach S, Moist L, Lindsay RM: Management of anemia with quotidian hemodialysis. Am J Kidney Dis 2003;42(suppl):18–23.

7 Lindsay RM, Alhejaili F, Nesrallah G, Leitch R, Clement L, Heidenheim AP, et al: Calcium and phosphate balance with quotidian hemo-dialysis. Am J Kidney Dis 2003;42(suppl): 24–29.

8 Spanner E, Suri R, Heidenheim AP, Lindsay RM: The impact of quotidian hemodi-alysis on nutrition. Am J Kidney Dis 2003; 42(suppl):30–35.

9 Oreopoulos DG, Thodis E, Passadakis P, Vargemezis V: Home dialysis as a first option: a new paradigm. Int Urol Nephrol 2009;41:595–605.

10 Mailloux LU, Kapikian N, Napolitano B, Mossey RT, Bellucci AG, Wilkes BM, et al: Home hemodialysis: patient outcomes dur-ing a 24-year period of time from 1970 through 1993. Adv Ren Replace Ther 1996;3: 112–119.

11 Woods JD, Port FK, Stannard D, Blagg CR, Held PJ: Comparison of mortality with home hemodialysis and center hemodialy-sis: a national study. Kidney Int 1996;49: 1464–1470.

12 McGregor DO, Buttimore AL, Lynn KL: Home hemodialysis: excellent survival at less cost, but still underutilized. Kidney Int 2000; 57:2654–2655.

13 Devereux RB, Reichek N: Echocardiographic determination of left ventricular mass in man. Anatomic validation of the method. Circulation 1977;55:613–618.

14 Suri RS, Nesrallah GE, Mainra R, Garg AX, Lindsay RM, Greene T, et al: Daily hemo-dialysis: a systematic review. Clin J Am Soc Nephrol 2006;1:33–42.

15 Pierratos A, Ouwendyk M, Francoeur R, Vas S, Raj DS, Ecclestone AM, et al: Nocturnal hemodialysis: three-year experience. J Am Soc Nephrol 1998;9:859–868.

16 Chan CT, Jain V, Picton P, Pierratos A, Floras JS: Nocturnal hemodialysis increases arterial baroreflex sensitivity and compliance and normalizes blood pressure of hypertensive patients with end-stage renal disease. Kidney Int 2005;68:338–344.

17 Fagugli RM, Pasini P, Pasticci F, Ciao G, Cicconi B, Buoncristiani U: Effects of short daily hemodialysis and extended standard hemodialysis on blood pressure and cardiac hypertrophy: a comparative study. J Nephrol 2006;19:77–83.

18 Bergman A, Fenton SS, Richardson RM, Chan CT: Reduction in cardiovascular related hospitalization with nocturnal home hemodialysis. Clin Nephrol 2008;69:33–39.

19 Culleton BF, Walsh M, Klarenbach SW, Mortis G, Scott-Douglas N, Quinn RR, et al: Effect of frequent nocturnal hemodialysis vs. conventional hemodialysis on left ventricular mass and quality of life: a randomized con-trolled trial. JAMA 2007;298:1291–1299.

20 London GM: Vascular disease and athero-sclerosis in uremia. Blood Purif 2001;19: 139–142.

21 Chan CT: Cardiovascular effects of frequent intensive hemodialysis. Semin Dial 2004;17: 99–103.

22 Silberberg JS, Barre PE, Prichard SS, Sniderman AD: Impact of left ventricular hypertrophy on survival in end-stage renal disease. Kidney Int 1989;36:286–290.

23 Zoccali C, Benedetto FA, Mallamaci F, Tripepi G, Giacone G, Stancanelli B, et al: Left ventricular mass monitoring in the fol-low-up of dialysis patients: prognostic value of left ventricular hypertrophy progression. Kidney Int 2004;65:1492–1498.

24 Foley RN, Parfrey PS, Kent GM, Harnett JD, Murray DC, Barre PE: Long-term evolu-tion of cardiomyopathy in dialysis patients. Kidney Int 1998;54:1720–1725.

25 Neves PL, Silva AP, Bernardo I: Elderly patients in chronic hemodialysis: risk factors for left ventricular hypertrophy. Am J Kidney Dis 1997;30:224–228.

 Kojima·Hoshi·Watanabe·Takenaka·Suzuki

26 Foley RN, Herzog CA, Collins AJ: Blood pressure and long-term mortality in United States hemodialysis patients: USRDS Waves 3 and 4 Study. Kidney Int 2002;62:1784–1790.

27 Szczech LA, Reddan DN, Klassen PS, Coladonato J, Chua B, Lowrie EG, et al: Interactions between dialysis-related volume exposures, nutritional surrogates and mortality among ESRD patients. Nephrol Dial Transplant 2003;18:1585–1591.

28 Foley RN, Parfrey PS, Sarnak MJ: Clinical epidemiology of cardiovascular disease in chronic renal disease. Am J Kidney Dis 1998; 32(suppl 3):S112–S119.

29 Block GA, Port FK: Re-evaluation of risks associated with hyperphosphatemia and hyperparathyroidism in dialysis patients: recommendations for a change in management. Am J Kidney Dis 2000;35:1226–1237.

30 Melamed ML, Eustace JA, Plantinga L, Jaar BG, Fink NE, Coresh J, et al: Changes in serum calcium, phosphate, and PTH and the risk of death in incident dialysis patients: a longitudinal study. Kidney Int 2006;70: 351–357.

31 Toussaint N, Boddington J, Simmonds R, Waldron C, Somerville C, Agar J: Calcium phosphate metabolism and bone mineral density with nocturnal hemodialysis. Hemodial Int 2006;10:280–286.

32 Kooienga L: Phosphorus balance with daily dialysis. Semin Dial 2007;20:342–345.

33 Ayus JC, Mizani MR, Achinger SG, Thadhani R, Go AS, Lee S: Effects of short daily versus conventional hemodialysis on left ventricular hypertrophy and inflammatory markers: a prospective, controlled study. J Am Soc Nephrol 2005;16:2778–2788.

34 Thunberg BJ, Swamy AP, Cestero RV: Cross-sectional and longitudinal nutritional measurements in maintenance hemodialysis patients. Am J Clin Nutr 1981;34:2005–2012.

35 Marckmann P: Nutritional status of patients on hemodialysis and peritoneal dialysis. Clin Nephrol 1988;29:75–78.

36 Kaysen GA, Schoenfeld PY: Albumin homeostasis in patients undergoing continuous ambulatory peritoneal dialysis. Kidney Int 1984;25:107–114.

37 Kaysen GA, Rathore V, Shearer GC, Depner TA: Mechanisms of hypoalbuminemia in hemodialysis patients. Kidney Int 1995;48: 510–516.

Hiromichi Suzuki, MD, PhD
Department of Nephrology, Saitama Medical University
38 Moroyama-machi, Iruma-gun
Saitama 350-0495 (Japan)
Tel. +81 49276 1620, E-Mail iromichi@saitama-med.ac.jp

Suzuki H (ed): Home Dialysis in Japan.
Contrib Nephrol. Basel, Karger, 2012, vol 177, pp 178–183

Development of a Nanotechnology-Based Dialysis Device

Yoshihiko Kanno[a] · Norihisa Miki[b]

[a]Apheresis and Dialysis Center, Department of Medicine, and [b]Department of Mechanical Engineering, Keio University, Tokyo, Japan

Abstract

Over 300,000 patients who need renal replacement therapy in our country are struggling to cope with daily life restrictions and complications because of dialysis therapy. They have to spend 3 half days a week for hemodialysis therapy which accounts for 95% of all renal replacement therapies in Japan. Moreover, they also have to be afraid of many complications associated with dialysis. Although these complications mostly arise from the shortage of dialysis quantity, we have been unable to improve the hemodialysis therapy system using extracorporeal circulation. Recently, we clinically investigated long-term dialysis therapies – one was a home-dialysis system and the other a portable dialysis system. We have also developed a very small dialysis device using nanotechnology, considering an implantable artificial kidney instead of transplantation in the near future.

Dialysis therapy was clinically introduced in humans in the 1960s to avoid death from later renal failure. The hemodialysis (HD) technique was predominately developed in Japan and became one of the few areas to lead the world in this field. Now, 95% of approximately 300,000 patients with end-stage renal failure receive HD therapy in our country as opposed to peritoneal dialysis or renal transplantation [1]. Although in the 1960s, at the dawn of dialysis therapy, it was been able to extend a patient's life for only several months, it is now not unusual that patients receiving HD can live 30 years or more due to technological advances.

Problems in the Present Dialysis System

Although the current system of HD is almost completed, there are several points that need improvement. Firstly, patients receiving HD struggle to cope with life restrictions. Generally, HD therapy requires bed rest for 3–4 h afterwards, vessel puncture, and hospital/clinic visits 3 times/week for a lifetime. A strict restriction on food and water intake is also necessary [2] because general dialysis therapy cannot remove enough water and body waste to allow the patient to drink and eat freely. Secondly, several severe complications due to a shortage of dialysis quantity occur in patients receiving HD over a long period of time, e.g. mineral bone disease, amyloidosis, calcification of major and peripheral vessels [3–6]. These complications have been well investigated but the absolute shortage of dialysis devices cannot be improved as long as we use the present therapeutic system. Thirdly, repeated contractions and extensions in the short term damage the vessels resulting in cardiovascular events which are the most common cause of death in HD patients. This is also due to the therapeutic system where a dialysis device removes the water and waste of 48 h in 3–4 h. These problems show a poor prognosis in HD patients where the 5-year survival is below 60%, even in Japan [1]. It is thought that the only strategy would be to increase dialysis in patients to improve these problems. Adding to these medical problems, there are also social problems such as infectious waste. In our country, dialyzers and other circuit systems are used only once. About 0.2 m³ of infectious waste is produced 3 times/week per person and its cost of disposal is about USD 80.

To the present day, there are only a few ways of increasing the amount of dialysis. Continuous renal replacement therapy (CRRT) was established in 1977 by Kramer et al. [7] who controlled body fluid balance using hemofiltration technology by the difference in arterial and venous pressures in critical patients. This method improved the prognosis of critically ill patients with mainly acute kidney injury. By minimizing the extracorporeal volume in HD, it might be possible to avoid the fall in blood pressure during the session. However, it also has to extend the treatment time to compensate for the reduction of dialysis efficiency per hour. This method would be useful to ensure that dialysis efficacies are sufficient enough for the patient without a critical status by continuing dialysis 48 h for 2 days. Actually, this method cannot be used in patients receiving usual HD, because CRRT requires patients to be connected to an extracorporeal circulation system, which means that patients receiving CRRT cannot leave their bed lifelong.

Idea and Clinical Investigation of Portable Dialysis System

The idea of portable HD using a smaller dialysis system was suggested from the dawn of clinical dialysis therapy [8]. Although this attractive idea has been considered difficult because of technical reasons, a wearable kidney module has finally been clinically investigated [9]. Using this system, patients could walk around carrying a miniaturized dialysis system which worked 24 h, 365 days. One of the technical developments of this system is that the adsorbent could recycle dialysate so that the patients could leave their bed in the dialysis room. The dream of every dialysis physician might come true with such an outstanding system, however several problems still exist, for example it needs deep vein access where it can draw blood into the extracorporeal circuit system. Patients have to put the blood tube around their body to avoid the risk of hemorrhage. Blood access is still one of the most serious problems when humans need extracorporeal circulation therapy.

Microdialyzer Using Nanotechnology

General interest in nanotechnology beyond biology started in the late 1990s in the area of drug delivery, diagnosis and the properties of nanoscale objects and materials [10]. In the area of dialysis, Ronco et al. [11] began to apply these new technologies to membranes and adsorbents. In fact, the adsorbent used in their wearable kidney system is a product using such nanotechnology [9].

We also developed a microfilter in 2007 utilizing a porous polyethersulfone (PES) membrane with nanopores [12]. As shown in figure 1, PES, polyvinylpyrrolidone (PVP), and 1-methyl-2-pyrrolidone (NMP) acting as solute, solvent and additives respectively were mixed and kept in a dark environment at room temperature for about 48 h to form transparent casting solutions. A nanoporous membrane was formed by the wet-phase inversion method as shown in figure 1 (left column). First, the casting solution was poured into a shallow bath at room temperature and squeegeed with a glass chip or a glass rod. Immediately after the solution became steady, the immersed solution was placed into the gelatin medium where a white layer of membrane was noticed appearing in the shallow bath. The PES membranes formed were kept in distilled water at room temperature for more than 24 h in order to remove the remaining PVP for further use. The sizes of the pores formed in the membrane were 2–5 nm.

The chamber layer was fabricated by deep wet etching. Ti plates (99.5%), 200 µm thick, were cut into pieces of 24 × 24 mm^2. The wide channel structures on these Ti layers were patterned using a positive photoresist AZ4260 (AZ Electric Materials). The measured geometrical parameters of the fabricated structural layer were tried in various scales. The Ti layers with wide channels were then bonded to the PES porous membranes using NMP, a solvent for PES. As illustrated in figure 1 (right column), a thin layer of NMP was prepared on a glass slide and was moved onto the surface of Ti layers by simple stamping. The PES membranes were then inserted between every second Ti layer immediately before the NMP evaporated. The polydimethylsiloxane cover layers were also bonded to the outside Ti layers by this method except that polydimethylsiloxane mortar was used instead of NMP. The assembled 9-unit microfilter (which means there were 9 pieces of PES porous membranes and 10 pieces of structural layers) is shown in figure 1. Inside the 9-unit microfilter there were 10

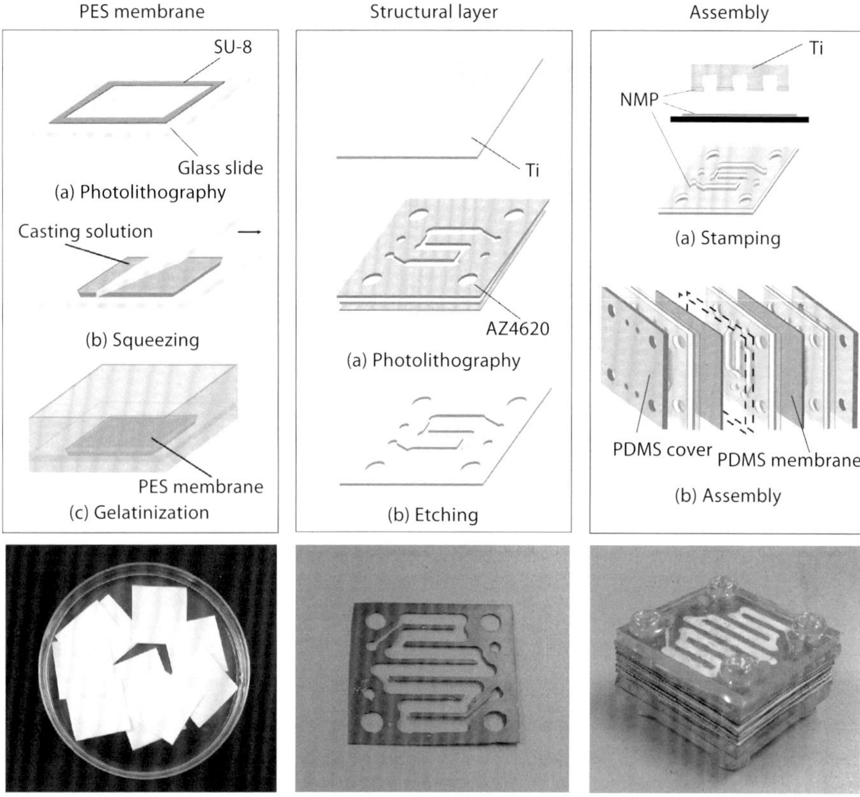

Fig. 1. Fabrication process of the nanotechnological dialysis device: *left:* preparing PES membrane using photolithography; *center:* preparing a structural layer by titanium plate; *right:* combining PES membrane and titanium plate to the device.

chambers divided into two groups: 5 for the flow of the analyte and 5 for the flow of the dialysate. To avoid leakage, the assembled device was compressed slightly and fastened in that compressed form with four plastic screws. To keep the PES membranes soaked, the device was kept in distilled water before being used in experiments.

The device we developed for dialysis was also evaluated for its function. The theoretical and experimental results of in vitro diffusing rates in each diffusing unit by flow rate of the blood phase in the 9-unit microfilter are shown in figure 2. The experimental results agreed well with the calculated theoretical values of all cases with low and high dialysate flow ratios. However, even when the rate of dialysate flow was 100 times higher than the rate of the blood phase (n = 100), which is reasonably considered as the maximum value, the diffusing rate of urea was still extremely close to that in the 'n = 1' case, which indicated that the diffusion rates could indeed be increased by increasing the flow of the dialysate phase. On the other hand, even the dialysate flow had

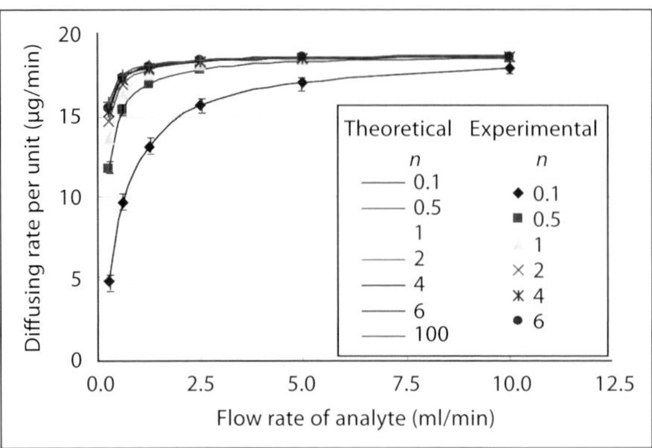

Fig. 2. Diffusing rate by flow rates of the blood phase. Theoretical and experimental results were agreed in all dialysate/blood ratios.

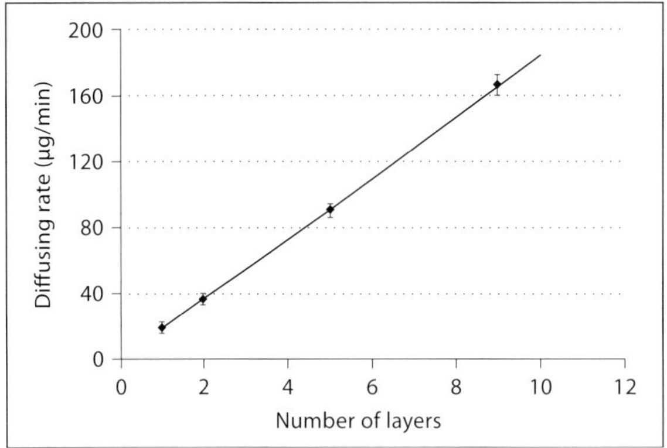

Fig. 3. Permeation of NaCl mixed with FITC dextrans of different sizes at a flow rate of 20 µl min^{-1}. The diffusing rate increased according to the number of layers added.

a much lower rate in the 'n = 0.1' case; the urea diffusion rate was 5% lower than the maximum value, which implied that even low-power pumps can be used to drive the dialysate phase in our device. The diffusing rates of urea by the number of layers in the devices are shown in figure 3. The rate of urea diffusion increased linearly with the increase of layers employed in the device at a rate of about 18 µg min^{-1} per diffusing unit. On the other hand, the FITC-dextran 70K, which is considered more or less the same size as the smallest protein albumin and larger than the pore size of the membranes, did not pass even only a little through the PES nanoporous membrane. Compared to the rate of urea removal by the human kidney, which is about 7.5 mg min^{-1}, it can be imagined that a 400-unit device, which is only about 40% the size

Kanno · Miki

of a human kidney, would be able to remove urea as fast as a human kidney does.

Thus our new dialysis device could remove enough urea from urea solution to use it in vivo. Considering its small size, it may be possible to implant this device into the human body instead of kidney transplantation, which is always short of a donor kidney. Although it may be difficult to supply dialyzate to the device in vitro, the arteriovenous hemofiltration mode without dialyzate [13] can remove enough water and waste to survive. If the function is not good enough, we are sure that the patient receiving HD can avoid one or two dialysis sessions a week. In the near future, implant dialysis systems will come into wide use as ideal home-dialysis devices.

References

1 Nakai S, Suzuki K, Masakane I, et al: Overview of regular dialysis treatment in Japan as of 31 December 2008. Ther Apher Dial 2010;14:505–540.

2 Kanno Y, Sasaki S, Suzuki H: Nutritional assessment by a new method for patients with renal disease. Contrib Nephrol. Basel, Karger, 2007, vol 155, pp 29–39.

3 Locatelli F, Pozzoni P, Del Vecchio L: Anemia and heart failure in chronic kidney disease. Semin Nephrol 2005;25:392–396.

4 Pozzoni P, Pozzi M, Del Vecchio L, Locatelli F: Epidemiology and prevention of cardio-vascular complication in chronic kidney disease patients. Semin Nephrol 2004;24: 417–422.

5 Eckardt KU: Anaemia in end-stage renal disease: pathophysiological considerations. Nephrol Dial Transplant 2001;16(suppl 7): 2–8.

6 Farrell J, Bastani B: Beta-2-microglobulin amyloidosis in chronic dialysis patients: a case report and review of the literature. J Am Soc Nephrol 1997;8:509–514.

7 Kramer P, Matthaei D, Rieger J, Scheler F: A new automatic haemofiltration machine with continuously monitored fluid balance. Proc Eur Dial Transplant Assoc 1977;14:613–617.

8 Stephens RL, Jacobsen SC, Atkin-thor E, Kolff W: Portable/wearable artificial kidney (WAK) – initial evaluation. Proc Eur Dial Transplant Assoc 1976;12:511–518.

9 Davenport A, Gura V, Ronco C, Beizai M, Ezon C, Rambod E: A wearable haemo-dialysis device for patients with end-stage renal failure: a pilot study. Lancet 2007;370: 2005–2010.

10 Thrall JH: Nanotechnology and medicine. Radiology 2004;230:315–318.

11 Nissenson AR, Ronco C: Nanotechnology and dialysis. Int J Artif Organs 2004;27:3–5.

12 Gu Y, Miki N: A microfilter utilizing a polyethersulfone porous membrane with nanopores. J Micromech Microeng 2007;17: 2308–2315.

13 Murisasco A, Reynier JP, Ragon A, et al: Continuous arteriovenous hemofiltration in a wearable device to treat end-stage renal disease. ASAIO Trans 1986;32:567–571.

Yoshihiko Kanno, MD, PhD
Apheresis and Dialysis Center
School of Medicine, Keio University
35 Shinanomachi Shinjuku, Tokyo 160-8582 (Japan)
Tel. +81 33353 1211, E-Mail kannoyh@a3.keio.jp

Author Index

Subject Index